Endometriosis

To all women with endometriosis, may your voices be heard so that future generations will have real hope of answers, an easier diagnosis, better treatments and even a cure, and to the healthcare professionals who dedicate their careers to helping women with endometriosis – despite the many challenges – thank you for not giving up

Endometriosis

The Experts' Guide to Treat, Manage and Live Well with Your Symptoms

Professor Andrew Horne and Carol Pearson

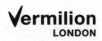

Vermilion
LONDON

1 3 5 7 9 10 8 6 4 2

Vermilion, an imprint of Ebury Publishing,
20 Vauxhall Bridge Road,
London SW1V 2SA

Vermilion is part of the Penguin Random House group of companies
whose addresses can be found at global.penguinrandomhouse.com

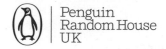

Penguin
Random House
UK

Copyright © Andrew Horne and Carol Pearson 2018

Andrew Horne and Carol Pearson have asserted their right to be
identified as the authors of this Work in accordance with
the Copyright, Designs and Patents Act 1988

First published in the United Kingdom by Vermilion in 2018

www.penguin.co.uk

A CIP catalogue record for this book is available from
the British Library

ISBN 9781785041471

Typeset in 11/15.8 pt Sabon LT Std
by Integra Software Services Pvt. Ltd, Pondicherry

Printed and bound in Great Britain by Clays Ltd, St Ives PLC

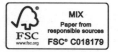

Penguin Random House is committed to a sustainable
future for our business, our readers and our planet.
This book is made from Forest Stewardship Council®
certified paper.

Contents

Foreword

Endometriosis is not straightforward. It is a disease where cells similar to those lining the womb grow elsewhere in the body. Where they grow, how much they grow, how deep they grow, and what they interfere with will vary from person to person – and so each individual with the disease experiences a different range of symptoms, and to a different severity. Despite affecting 10 per cent of women of reproductive age – 1.5 million in the UK, 176 million worldwide – there is no cure, and treatments are not always helpful and can come with risks or side effects.

The average length of time to get a diagnosis is, shockingly, 7.5 years. Being an average this masks a significant range   from women who receive great support and are diagnosed in just a few months because their GP suspects endometriosis early on and navigates the route to diagnosis efficiently, through to women for whom diagnosis takes 15 years or more. Before a diagnosis, effective treatment options cannot easily be offered. Before a diagnosis, a woman may be told her symptoms are 'normal', may be misdiagnosed with another condition, or may even be told her symptoms are 'in her head'. They may miss work or education, unable to put a name to their 'problems', hampering their careers – endometriosis costs the UK economy an estimated £8.2bn a year in treatment, loss of work and healthcare costs. This is no way for women to be treated in the 21st century.

There is no doubt that endometriosis can sometimes be a challenge to diagnose and to treat. Symptoms are shared by a range of other conditions – chronic pelvic pain can be associated with pelvic inflammatory disease, fibroids, irritable bowel syndrome and painful bladder syndrome, to name just a few, as well as due to endometriosis. Endometriosis doesn't always show up on scans and the only definitive diagnosis at present is through surgery, so it makes sense to rule out other conditions first if that can be done less invasively. But endometriosis should be considered when a woman has one or more symptoms, and sadly that doesn't always happen.

There are steps that we can take to significantly reduce diagnosis times and improve the treatments women are offered. Raising awareness of menstrual health and what's normal as part of education in schools, so no-one puts up with years of pain and other problems thinking it's 'normal'. Raising public awareness – after all, this affects 10 per cent of women irrespective of race or socioeconomic background, so shouldn't everyone know about it? We need tools and guidance to help GPs, as well as wider availability of resources to treat women effectively, so women don't have to wait months – sometimes years – for surgery they very much need. Investment in research is vital to find answers about what causes endometriosis and effective treatments.

Vitally important, we need to support women with endometriosis, or who suspect they might have it, to ensure they have the information and support they need to help manage their condition. And this is where this book comes in; we hope it will provide help to women, and all those that support them, to navigate through their journey with endometriosis.

Many thanks to Carol Pearson and Professor Andrew Horne, our authors. Together they have produced this expert guide through their knowledge and many years of experience working with and championing the needs of women with endometriosis, bringing together the voices of patients and clinicians.

Emma Cox,
CEO, Endometriosis UK,
2017

Introduction

Imagine that you spend months – no, let's make that years, maybe many years – in pain, excruciating pain, but you think, or are told, that what you're going through is normal. You wrack your brain for answers. It doesn't add up. Something is not right! You know it, but others can't see it, even people that you're really close to.

You seek help, seeing one doctor, then another, you try this drug and then that one, but you're not getting better .... you get referred to a hospital and the same routine starts over again. You have one invasive test or scan followed by another, and still no answers. Finally, someone operates ... And, one day you are told that you have a disease called 'endometriosis'.

But you haven't heard of it – nor has your partner, your mother or your friend. Later, you're back at work or college and though you tell them it still hurts, no one understands. You have more surgery – aren't you better yet, everyone says? No, you're not. You start more treatment, have more surgery, you feel a bit better but then it comes back again .... and so it goes on.

If you were told that this was a disease that affected one in 10 women, and yet this story still goes on all over the world today, you would be deeply shocked. How can this happen? Women's bodies – women's problems – have been so taboo and this silence has cost society.

In the many years that we have both been involved supporting or looking after women with endometriosis, we have heard this story literally hundreds of times. The stories invariably involve women who have experienced a delay in diagnosis; they often involve women seeing a whole range of healthcare professionals and having an array of tests and several – maybe even many – surgeries. They involve many years of suffering, sometimes with a positive ending, but not always.

Our book provides up-to-date information on endometriosis and the latest treatments available, linked to real stories of many women with endometriosis. We want you to hear about the stories of these women – women who have often hidden their suffering and tried desperately to live 'normal' lives. How the women coped, what were the highs and lows, what impact did this disease have on them – their relationships, their fertility, their careers and their hopes and dreams? We want to show you not just the women behind this disease but also their partners, their family members – and the GPs, gynaecologists, nurses, and allied healthcare practitioners who work so hard to treat women with endometriosis, because their stories are part of that fabric too. These women – they could be you, or your partner, sister, daughter or mother, or they could be your patient, sitting patiently telling you again that they are in pain – whoever they are, they must be listened to.

While researching for this book, we conducted in-depth interviews with women with endometriosis and a wide range of clinicians. We are deeply grateful to all of them. Through these interviews, we listened to over 50 hours of experiences from a range of different perspectives, amounting to some 300,000 words solely on endometriosis and the care of women with this disease. Despite being involved in the field of endometriosis for many years, analysing these interviews revealed many surprises.

In choosing to talk, the women in this book made themselves vulnerable. It was very hard for them to relive elements of their stories that they had long filed away in their memories, and we will be for ever indebted to them that they had the courage to do this to help other women and to help people generally understand how endometriosis affects us and our society today. We also want to pay tribute to the clinicians whom we spoke to who treat women with endometriosis – their path is also not an easy one at all. This is no straightforward disease, either to diagnose or treat. Without their tenacity and knowledge, women with endometriosis would be far worse off.

Professor Andrew Horne and Carol Pearson,
2017

A note on terminology

When we talk about women in this book, we refer to our many years of experience working with women with endometriosis plus the series of in-depth interviews we conducted prior to starting writing. We could not hope to replicate even a fraction of all we've been told but hope that the main themes are captured. When we refer to 'clinicians', we similarly refer to the many clinicians in diverse clinical roles with whom we have worked and those with whom we conducted similar interviews.

Endometriosis is a gynaecological disease – which means it's related to the female reproductive system – when cells similar (but not the same) as those that line the utcrus (womb), grow in other places. These usually grow in the pelvis but on occasion grow elsewhere in the body. These areas of abnormal tissue respond to hormones and are thought to 'bleed' on a monthly basis, causing symptoms such as pain and resulting in scarring and inflammation. Endometriosis is not cancer, nor is it an infection. The cause of endometriosis remains unknown.

These growths are commonly referred to as lesions and nodules, and occasionally implants. You may also hear the term endometrioma, which specifically refers to endometriosis in the ovary.

Symptoms of endometriosis vary, however, if you experience any of these it could be endometriosis:

- Pain: with periods, with sex or pelvic pain at other times of the month that interferes with everyday life.

- Bowel symptoms: e.g., diarrhoea, constipation and painful bowel movements.

- Bladder symptoms: e.g., pain when urinating.

- Fatigue.

- Difficulty getting pregnant.

Classification systems for endometriosis

This enigmatic, rather mysterious disease has been subject to various classification systems over the years, none of which are wholly satisfactory.

When we refer to superficial disease, we refer to disease that does not penetrate deeply into the surface of organs. Some classifications refer to this as 'minimal' or 'mild' disease, or disease stages 1 to 2. It may be in isolated areas or widespread.

When we refer to deep disease, we refer to deeper lesions. Some classifications refer to this as 'moderate' or 'severe' disease, or disease stage 3 or 4. Again, it may be in isolated areas or widespread. It may involve the ovaries, forming 'cysts' or 'endometriomas', sometimes referred to as 'chocolate cysts' and/or have penetrated organs, such as the bowel or bladder.

It is important to acknowledge upfront that none of these classifications describes in any way either the extent to which a woman experiences symptoms from this condition, or the level of disability. There is absolutely no discrimination. Deep disease can, on occasions, be silent and symptomless; superficial disease can be disabling, and vice versa.

A woman's anatomy

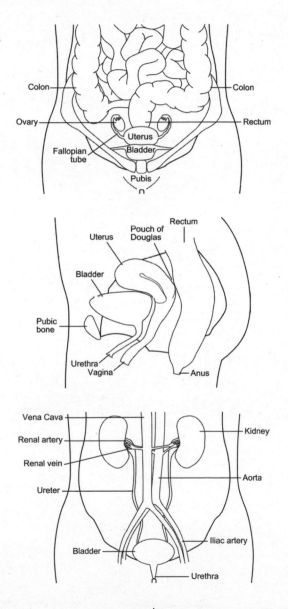

Chapter 1

Endometriosis: definition and diagnosis today

We live in an age transformed by the power of social media and technology: there have never been more ways to communicate, so quickly and efficiently. Thankfully, we also benefit from unprecedented openness – we can freely share our innermost thoughts, feelings and challenges if we want to – not just with our friends and family but also with complete strangers. We have seen this with many issues that have been previously stigmatised, including mental health and sexuality. We're seeing the start of a similar revolution on menstruation but there's still a way to go. So, why do we still shy away from 'female things'? Is there still an unspoken 'otherness' about being a woman, despite 49.5 per cent of the world's population being female? Unfortunately, for one in 10 women, who have this very misunderstood, poorly explained disease, endometriosis, the social movement has only just begun – and it couldn't have come a moment too soon. But what exactly is endometriosis?

The lowdown on endometriosis

It was like opening a door into another world that I had no clue how to navigate, who to talk to, how to get support, or get myself better. – Zoe

Endometriosis – or 'endo', as women with the condition often come to call it – is commonly considered to be a gynaecological disease, or a disease of the female pelvic organs. But on another level, it is also a system-wide hormonal disease that strikes right at the cellular level, because endometriosis occurs when cells that act like those that line the womb (uterus) are found elsewhere, usually in the pelvis, in places where they are extremely unwelcome: on the lining of the peritoneal wall (the inside lining of the abdomen and pelvis), in the ovaries, in the vagina, on or even in the bowel or bladder, and sometimes, rarely, in far-flung corners of the body, such as the diaphragm, the covering of the heart (pericardium), the lungs (causing a cyclical cough, or cyclical coughing up of blood), in abdominal scars, including the navel, or belly button. In exceptionally rare cases, it has even been known to present in men.

So what happens then? Well, we know that endometriosis is a disease that grows in response to hormones – principally oestrogen – coming from the ovaries. Oestrogen is the hormone that causes your womb lining to thicken each month. The endometriosis tissue responds to the body's oestrogen and likely bleeds 'internally' with no place to go. Over time, this monthly internal bleeding can lead to inflammation and scarring – referred to as 'adhesions' – that can cause surfaces within the pelvis to stick together.

The misplaced endometriosis tissue may develop its own blood supply to help it grow, and a nerve supply to communicate with the brain, which is one possible reason why some women with endometriosis may suffer from such debilitating pain. But women with endometriosis can also suffer from a wide range of other symptoms and issues, such as a range of digestive symptoms (constipation, diarrhoea, nausea and IBS type symptoms), painful sex, subfertility, pelvic pain either persistently throughout the month or at certain times, and fatigue. Strangely, not every woman with endometriosis gets pain but many of them do – and we could write a book alone on the pain associated with endometriosis. When thinking about the symptoms of endometriosis, it can be helpful to look at where all the organs are located in a woman's pelvis. There's a useful illustration of this at the start of this book (see page xxi).

Why do women get endometriosis?

Theories abound as to why women get endometriosis and what causes it – the truth is we do not know conclusively, as yet, why some women get it. But we can describe some of the characteristics of it that will help us to understand it a little better.

Genetics

Above all, we know that you are more likely to have endometriosis if you have a relative with it. But, in truth, the genetics of endometriosis is complex and remains unexplained. Most researchers feel that endometriosis is inherited by what is termed as 'a polygenic/multifactorial mode', which means that it is caused by a combination of genes and the environment. Yet there are a number of factors that specifically make it difficult to determine the exact 'mode' of inheritance of endometriosis.

First and foremost is the fact that endometriosis can only be diagnosed invasively by surgery. This can result in under-reporting of patients with the disease since the diagnosis relies on an invasive test.

Another issue is that endometriosis may not actually be one disease but a number of similar diseases that are currently grouped together under the definition of 'endometriosis', as evidenced by the different sites in the body where it can be found. So there is, as yet, no 'genetic' test for endometriosis. Many of the women we spoke to talked of their own mum's sufferings, or that of other family members who perhaps never realised they had endometriosis.

I think my mum definitely had endo but she wasn't diagnosed. Her sister did have endo and was luckily diagnosed. – Lucy

Sampson's theory

Putting genetic factors aside, another widely accepted and supported explanation for why women develop endometriosis is 'Sampson's theory', first put forward in the 1920s by gynaecologist Dr John Sampson, that suggests it occurs due to 'retrograde menstruation'. This is where some of the blood and cells that are shed from the womb lining during a period pass backwards up through the Fallopian tubes into the pelvis and stick to the pelvic cavity wall instead of leaving the womb through the vagina as part of the monthly period. Yet we know that nearly 90 per cent of women experience retrograde menstruation and most women with retrograde menstruation do not end up with endometriosis. Because of this, studies to date have focused on differences in the womb lining of women with endometriosis and researchers are now investigating whether the pelvic wall lining (peritoneum) plays a role in the establishment of the condition, or whether it is altered in women with endometriosis.

The newborn menstruation hypothesis

We also know from research that endometriosis cells have been found in the foetus, which supports the theory that the disease process is laid down in some women from the start of their lives. The lining of the womb in a newborn baby can show signs of activity immediately after birth and, in some cases, show changes similar to those seen at menstruation in women. So, the womb in a newborn baby is capable of shedding its lining, yes, 'menstruating'. Indeed, visible vaginal bleeding occurs in one in 20 newborn female babies. And what's fascinating is that endometriosis has been seen in a newborn baby – possibly due to plugging of the womb at the level of the cervix, the womb outlet – leading to a backward, or retrograde, flux of the blood and cells contained in menstrual debris. These findings are causing researchers to speculate that endometriosis, especially in children and young adolescents, could originate from retrograde bleeding soon after birth.

Other hypotheses

Some researchers think that endometriosis could be an immune system problem or that a local hormonal imbalance enables the endometrial-like tissue to take root and grow after it is pushed out of the uterus. Others believe that in some women, certain pelvic wall or abdominal cells mistakenly turn into endometrial cells (metaplasia). These same cells are the ones responsible for the growth of a woman's reproductive organs in the embryonic stage. It's believed that something in the woman's genetic makeup, or something she's exposed to in the environment later in life, changes those cells so that they turn into endometrial tissue outside the uterus. There's also some thinking that damage to cells that line the pelvis from a previous infection can lead to endometriosis.

Despite these theories we still have unanswered questions, questions that research still needs to answer. Most experts agree that there are many factors that may all have a role in the development of endometriosis, including genetic factors, retrograde menstruation, metaplasia, immunological and hormonal reasons.

We've looked at what endometriosis is and some of the theories about why women get it, let's now take a look at one of the challenges of this disease: getting a diagnosis.

Diagnosis: when is 'normal' not normal?

Most young women have some pain and discomfort, leading up to, during and after their period. This is normal, and most girls get told that their periods will calm down in a couple of years as hormone levels become more settled; for most girls they will. But 'period pain' should not be so bad that you cannot get up, go to school, college or work, or carry on with your normal life. If your pain is interfering with everyday activities, at any age, it is not normal.

The taboo that requires a woman's common bodily functions to remain largely unspoken of, is a stumbling block when it comes to diagnosing and treating endometriosis. But let's start at the very first challenge facing women – and probably the most fundamental issue for endometriosis – the notion that period pain is 'normal'. How can people know and distinguish between 'normal pain' and pain that is a problem, pain that might indicate disease may be present? How do we know what is 'normal?'

Let's call this first stage 'the unknown unknown': quite simply, we just don't know what we don't know. For many with endometriosis, the first stumbling block is this: that the perception of women's pain is quite clearly embedded in our society and that starts with education at home, often by other women, so, unfortunately for some teenagers, their 'norm' was also their mother's or their grandmother's pain. Amy explains: 'I was in one of those families where my mum and my nan said, "It was really bad for us as well, we're just unlucky as a family."'

How deeply ironic for a disease that has a hereditary component that the pain and disease of some mothers and grandmothers – who very sadly may have had the disease and not even have known it – should be one of the reasons why women may delay seeking help for pain.

If we expect women to be in pain, how do we break that down? How do we dispel the myth that pain is inseparable from having a period, and secondly, how do we help people to understand the important – and early – indicators of this common disease, endometriosis? Perhaps a good place to start would be in health education in schools, but even there, as Preena explains, there is no mention of common diseases that affect periods, such as endometriosis. 'I had no idea about any of these things when I was young, and I think many young girls suffer from it but unfortunately they're not told about it, either at school or university.'

So, let's move to stage two, the 'known unknown': you're becoming aware that there is a problem, but have absolutely no idea what's wrong, you just know things are definitely not 'normal' with your periods. Perhaps over-the-counter pain relief isn't enough to help manage your symptoms and maybe you have even already been to see your GP. At this stage, your symptoms may cause you to take time off work, or to miss school.

Whatever it is, when we asked women to talk us through their journeys with endometriosis, many of them started by talking about the challenges they faced early on as a teenager, even if they weren't diagnosed with endometriosis until many years later.

Early years with endometriosis

Endometriosis symptoms may be experienced at any age, ranging from when a girl reaches puberty to menopause. However, it can be especially difficult for those who suffer significantly when they are still at school, and unfortunately a myth persists that teenagers don't get endometriosis. Sophie's friend would take her to the medical room when she had her period as the pain she experienced made her vomit 'It was very embarrassing, because every time my friend would go back to the classroom, the teacher would ask what was wrong and my friend would say, "oh it's tummy pains again", and all the pupils would laugh and think I was really weak and not coping with period pains.'

Beth experienced a lot of fatigue. 'Everyone thought I was lazy because I missed quite a lot of school every month. They would get my mum in and said I wouldn't pass my exams, and this is coming from an A-star student. So there was an obvious disconnect with how people saw me and how tired I was feeling, from doctors, teachers, the school nurse, everyone.'

How bizarre is it that we do not routinely talk to young women about knowing what may not be 'normal' and the symptoms of endometriosis? In most countries, there is still limited education about menstrual health, what's normal and what is not, and the subject of endometriosis is barely touched upon, if it is raised at all. And even worse – how awful is it that we potentially leave women to suffer for years and years as a result?

During this stage – which could last a few months or for many years – women are on their way to getting help, even if this is frustratingly slow sometimes. They're seeing doctors, sometimes quite a few of them. This part of the 'known unknown' is very tricky – they're entering a world of knowledge and possibility but there is often stark inconsistency of diagnoses and advice. Of course, no two women with endometriosis are the same and there is a vast range of symptoms, but there are two very key people in this stage: the GP and the gynaecologist. We'll take a detailed look at their roles in Chapter 3, The right care in the right place for you.

Information on symptoms

Let's get back to the actual disease itself, because the symptoms of it are a whole story in themselves, and one of the reasons why endometriosis can be so hard to identify. The long diagnosis time for endometriosis isn't just about the lack of information for teenage girls. When it comes to symptoms and subsequent tests, we're entering an even more challenging arena where women and clinicians need to work together to find answers.

For a start, we know the symptoms may or may not correlate to the severity of disease. Rather confusingly, 'superficial', 'mild', 'peritoneal' or 'stage 1' disease, which may involve a few spots of endometriosis in one or two areas, or spread across the inside of the pelvis, may cause persistently disabling symptoms, whilst some women with deep or severe disease may not necessarily experience symptoms that are as debilitating.

We know this conundrum and all we can do is face it and be honest. There is simply no pattern or explanation as to why symptoms are so variable and also why there are so many different symptoms. We should also note that some of these symptoms overlap with many other diseases, some of which women with endometriosis may also have, which rather complicates the situation.

If there is one thing that has frustrated women with this disease, it is probably this alone: that it may have taken an inordinate amount of time for unpleasant, sometimes disabling symptoms to be pinned down to a cause, and perhaps even to be taken seriously. Unfortunately, a large number of women are told a whole bunch of things that turn out, with hindsight, to be not quite right – on top of this, a huge number of tests may be endured and a lot of doctors may be seen along the way. Sadly, this can have a significant emotional impact. But let's take a closer look at the symptoms first.

Pain

Pain can be very hard to describe or even for others to understand, particularly when it relates to the inside of our bodies. For many women, endometriosis involves some level of pain, but this is certainly not the case for all women. However, for many women, pain is what defines endometriosis for them. Some women are in pain for a very long time before they seek help, whereas others seek help much quicker.

Women's pain may be constant, or cyclical, occurring each month during the same part of the menstrual cycle. This latter can be hard to monitor – unless actively pursuing pregnancy, women don't go around thinking, oh, I must be ovulating now ... so many women just think of it as 'intermittent'. Keeping a pain and symptoms diary (see page 47) to record what your symptoms are, when they occur and how they affect you, will help identify if there is any pattern to your pain. In either case, if the pain lasts over six months, it is referred to as chronic pain.

The women that we spoke to had lots of descriptions for their pain. Some only experienced pain during their periods, some at other specific times of the month, whereas others had pain throughout the month.

Zoe paints a picture of her pain: 'It's either an aching, dragging, heavy feeling from the waist down, or it's intensely sharp, stabbing. It feels like everything is going to fall out of you.' The feeling that everything is going to fall out is a description that quite a few women used.

If you have painful symptoms, how can you help others, and particularly healthcare practitioners, to understand this pain? First of all, it can help to explain how it affects your day-to-day life.

Pain that affects everyday activities

Part of describing the pain is explaining the effect of it – and this is key, because pain that causes girls to miss school or work indicates there may be an issue. Preena explains: 'I would have to miss days off school. The pain wasn't normal pain that my mum used to experience, this was fold-over on the bed in agony pain, taking the strongest ibuprofen possible.'

Pain that doesn't respond to over-the-counter painkillers from your pharmacist is an indication that you need to seek help from your doctor. And pain that affects everyday activities, such as sleeping, eating and sitting, should also be a strong indicator to seek medical attention. Madison describes this sort of pain: 'I couldn't concentrate, I didn't want to eat, I couldn't sleep for the pain, there was no position, sitting, lying, that was comfortable at all.'

Pain that causes other symptoms such as fainting, nausea and vomiting

Pain sometimes has a knock-on impact and causes other symptoms, such as fainting, nausea and vomiting.

Madison goes on to explain, 'the pain was so excruciating that it was almost like my body just shut down, I would pass out to deal with it and that was a recurring issue for quite a few years.'

Pain that has affected you for a long time

Some women that we talked to had pain right from when their periods started, maybe even before. Generally, teenage girls experiencing pelvic pain see their GP, who may prescribe analgesia or perhaps the oral contraceptive pill. And then it may be years, sometimes more than 10 years, before a woman for whatever reason decides to come off the pill and then, out of the blue, she's again hit with terrible pain.

Not every woman is in pain for years though. Emily's pain came on very quickly and severely, as she relates 'I couldn't lift a kettle with my right hand, I couldn't drive, massive, massive pain. Of course, I'd no idea what it was, it was really horrible, so the doctor asked lots of questions, sort of leaned on my stomach – I screamed in pain.'

Why am I in pain?

We don't know exactly why endometriosis lesions cause pain, but they do 'bleed' and result in scarring and inflammation and seem to form their own nerve and blood supply, which may explain this. The women we spoke to told us that they were given a variety of reasons for the pain they were experiencing before they were diagnosed with endometriosis. These include being told 'it will settle down', 'it's normal', 'it's a kidney infection', the list goes on.

The huge challenge for GPs is that a lot of teenage girls experience period pain, only some of which will be caused by endometriosis, so it can be very difficult for GPs to distinguish who to refer for tests. It can get even more confusing after that, as scans only show up certain types of endometriosis, so women often get discharged back to their GP with no answers.

There's one type of pain that we haven't mentioned so far, but this is very important when it comes to endometriosis: pain with sex. And when it comes to this, it can be very hard to raise it with anyone, let alone your doctor. But you can't afford to be shy about it.

Pain with intercourse

Okay, if there were problems explaining your pelvic pain, things just got a whole lot more difficult. How do you talk to your doctor about sex, where do you start?

> *I had lots of problems explaining to doctors that I have painful intercourse. They didn't really seem to understand and suggested it was due to different sizes of penises, or as I am quite small in height, it was down to me. Nobody really knew what to suggest except lubrication, and I found the conversation often got changed quickly.* – Sophie

When it comes to explaining your pain to your doctor, including pain with sex, it's best to be prepared:

- Remember to take copies of your pain and symptoms diary (see page 47)

- Book your appointment with a doctor that you are comfortable with, perhaps with one that has an interest in gynaecology or women's health

- If you're happy to do so, consider taking your partner or a family member with you for support

We'll take a closer look at painful sex in Chapter 4.

Pain in other parts of the body

One of the complicated aspects of endometriosis is that pain isn't always confined to the pelvis. It is another reason why it can be difficult to diagnose or understand. In particular, a number of women we interviewed experienced leg pain. A few of these women had endometriosis on the bowel, but not all of them.

Lucy's leg pain was quite disabling. 'I was prescribed amitriptyline and then nortriptyline [tricyclic antidepressants used to treat neuropathic pain] to try to help with the nerve pain. It was a constant "walking through water" feeling. Some days the leg pains were worse than the endo abdomen pains.'

Endometriosis that affects the 'obturator' nerve, a nerve that runs through the pelvis and supplies the inner thighs, can cause pain that radiates down the leg. Endometriosis can also cause leg pain when it affects the 'pudendal' nerve, a nerve that supplies part of the vagina and vulva.

Scarlett had terrible bowel pain which meant she couldn't sit down. She was later diagnosed with bowel endometriosis but the pain was very disruptive to her life. 'I couldn't go to work, I just had to lie down because I couldn't sit down in my job, most people would at least think it reasonable to be able to sit down, but no.'

We think of endometriosis as a gynaecological condition but it has a knock-on impact in quite a few other parts of the body. This is why functions such as walking or sitting can sometimes be seriously affected.

Bowel symptoms

Aside from pain, the women we interviewed were most bothered by a mixture of other symptoms that can broadly be classified as gastrointestinal – such as bloating, nausea, vomiting, diarrhoea and constipation. It's worth knowing that, when endometriosis affects other organs, the bowel is the one that is most commonly affected. But it's complicated. If the pain associated with endometriosis is often enigmatic (i.e., sometimes there's no pain with a lot of disease, but sometimes there is lots of pain with a little disease), then it's probably no surprise that the bowels are playing a similar game. So, women with endometriosis-related bowel disease (that's endometriosis growing on the surface of the bowel sometimes continuing all the way inside it and sometimes causing narrowing) may well experience bowel symptoms, but women who don't have bowel disease may unfortunately also experience bowel symptoms. Confused? Well, let's get the lowdown from these belligerent neighbours, the bowels.

Bloating

Let's first look at one of the troublesome and uncomfortable symptoms women identified – bloating. Sometimes, it was one of the main symptoms that resulted in women visiting their doctor, as Preena describes. 'When I was 17 years old, I noticed that I was getting very bloated to an extreme level, and I didn't know why. I looked like I was six months pregnant.' Preena ended up being diagnosed with a large ovarian cyst as part of her endometriosis. But why would this cause bloating? Well, unfortunately we don't fully understand why women with endometriosis experience uncomfortable bloating, but it is likely due to the inflammation from the endometriosis lesions.

Diarrhoea and constipation

Some women with endometriosis experience either diarrhoea or constipation, or both – again, whether endometriosis is on, in, or somewhere near the bowel may or may not affect how symptoms appear. Irrespective of this, the effects are the same: the bowels are not happy and the effects can be very debilitating.

So much so, that some of women were diagnosed with irritable bowel syndrome, or IBS, long before they received their diagnosis of endometriosis. And, confusingly, some women have both IBS and endometriosis. We're not yet able to explain fully whether the chances of having a diagnosis of IBS in women with endometriosis are due to misdiagnosis or true 'comorbidity' (i.e., that they are linked). Women with endometriosis may be operated on by gynaecologists with variable experience in the diagnosis and treatment of endometriosis. Even during laparoscopy (see page 24), some gynaecologists may fail to diagnose endometriosis. The diagnosis of bowel endometriosis may be even more difficult for a gynaecologist with limited experience in treating the condition. So, bowel endometriosis may remain undiagnosed even when a diagnosis of endometriosis elsewhere is made. This is relevant because intestinal endometriosis lesions may cause gastrointestinal symptoms and mimic IBS. It's perhaps not surprising then that women with superficial and/or ovarian endometriosis, and undiagnosed bowel endometriosis, are diagnosed with IBS and receive IBS treatments. The link between endometriosis and 'true' IBS remains to be proved.

Amy was very ill with bowel symptoms before she was diagnosed with endometriosis on the bowel. Her diarrhoea was so severe that she kept being hospitalised with it, as she explains 'I couldn't eat or drink without setting it off and I think I didn't eat for a week once, and then I couldn't drink either, so I ended up having to keep going into hospital to go on a drip.'

For Thea, it was the reverse – she started experiencing constipation with her periods and was very quickly diagnosed with endometriosis on the bowel. 'I was in agony for two or three days and I would try anything and everything, which never really seemed to make much difference. Once those three days had gone, I would then go to the toilet and then my bowel symptoms just went.'

Nicole continues to suffer IBS-type symptoms with her cycle, and finds this challenging. 'On my cycle, I have a week when it's really bad and then it calms down, and then another week where it flares up, then it calms down. At the moment, it's not so much the pain I get as the IBS. I can't control it.'

Some women find changing their diet helps them to manage both their pain and their bowel symptoms. We'll be looking at this further in Chapter 7: Adjusting life.

Bladder symptoms

Endometriosis affecting the bladder or urinary tract is less common. When it occurs, it is far more likely to affect the bladder than the upper part of the urinary tract, such as the kidneys. Sometimes it affects the ureters, the tubes taking urine from the kidneys to the bladder, but again this is relatively rare. A couple of the women we interviewed had endometriosis affecting their bladders, one of whom was Emily. She explains how her bladder is affected: 'When your bladder gets full, you can hold it, it's not that, it's not an incontinence feeling that I get. It starts to hurt and then after you empty, sometimes it hurts more.'

As with the bowel, the type of surgery involved for the bladder deserves special attention, so we'll look at this in Chapter 2: Making choices: treatment options.

Fatigue

One of the symptoms that often gets ignored but appears to be widespread is fatigue – and actually, the fact that women with endometriosis feel fatigued makes a great deal of sense. First of all, chronic pain can be exhausting and this may make dealing with even small tasks a challenge. Symptoms can disrupt sleep, meaning that you don't wake feeling refreshed and well. Also, endometriosis has a chronic inflammatory component to it, which means that there could be a knock-on effect on energy levels. We don't yet understand enough about why chronic inflammation causes fatigue, but it's thought that inflammation has an effect on the immune system and also on the brain and central nervous system, resulting in fatigue. If you then add on top of that the intriguing role of hormones, symptoms such as digestive problems and heavy bleeding, you've got the perfect combination of symptoms that cause persistent tiredness.

Preena struggles with this. 'I'm often very tired, even when I've done nothing to be tired for. Sometimes I get pain from my remaining ovary when I'm walking. It's just a mixture of things, it's just the feeling of not being 100 per cent all the time.'

Beth also suffers a lot with fatigue, which has affected her studies, but it was difficult to know how much was due to her symptoms and how much was due to her busy student life. 'During uni, things were getting worse but it was still just the monthly cycle of pain and bleeding, although fatigue did affect me more, but it's hard to tell because it's the first time in your life that you are truly independent and so it is really hard and you know, a degree is difficult and I had quite an active life, exercise, hobbies etc., so it was hard to tell how much was fatigue and how much was just doing a lot of stuff.'

As a final measure, then add on top of that loss of sleep from being in pain and trying to function in a world that doesn't always understand 'women's problems', then you've potentially got a recipe for exhaustion. Sophie says: 'It's when you've had days of non-stop pain, when you haven't slept because of pain or can't do anything because the pain is so bad or you have pain with fatigue. It becomes unbearable. Severe pain drains all your energy supplies so quickly.'

And it's no wonder that some women therefore described to us how often they simply just don't feel well, not 100 per cent. Imagine feeling like this for months on end, perhaps even longer. This is another symptom that can be so isolating.

Other symptoms

Although women with endometriosis often suffer from extremely painful periods, many women with endometriosis report that their period 'flow' is 'normal'. However some report irregular periods, prolonged bleeding, or premenstrual spotting. Others report that they experience heavy periods. We don't know if this is related to endometriosis or adenomyosis, where endometriosis-like cells grow in the muscle wall of the womb, which we'll talk about later in this chapter.

What we can say is that the women we spoke to reported a range of symptoms associated with bleeding, from bleeding after sex, which Nicole experienced: 'it was when I met my husband and I started bleeding after sex, so I thought "oh this is not right, this is not normal", so I went to the doctor', to the frustrations of irregular or heavy bleeding experienced by others. Preena constantly has to plan to take sanitary pads with her, because she never knows when she might start bleeding: 'I've literally got a constant supply of pads in my bag. You don't want to have to constantly worry about it, that you might bleed on the spot.'

Chloe used to pack extra underwear to take away on holiday with her and take additional clothes to work, in case she bled through them. She used to bleed for 23 days a month. 'I thought it was normal to take three sets of clothes to work, or to be on painkillers all the time. But then, suddenly, when it is not there, you suddenly go, oh. It was only last year that I stopped taking eight pairs of pants when I went away for two nights.'

The relationship between symptoms and types of endometriosis

When there's such a wide range of symptoms for this disease, you might well be asking if there's any correlation at all between symptoms and the type of endometriosis. As we mentioned right at the start, this is very tricky indeed. Why is this?

Well, for a start, there are women that have lots of tiny spots of disease scattered around their pelvis – called superficial or peritoneal disease – but we know that these can be women who have difficult, relentless symptoms. Remember that 'superficial' is used as a medical term to mean 'on the surface', not how it's used in everyday life, where 'superficial' often implies someone is shallow or phoney. This type of endometriosis can be hard to treat surgically because there may be small amounts but they can be widespread. Beth describes this type of endometriosis and explains why she remains in constant pain. 'I met with the specialist, and he said this is quite extensive endo. There is ten-plus years of scarring all over your peritoneum, bowel, bladder. There's little tiny dots, but everywhere, so I never really had to worry about needing a bit of bowel removed or anything like that, but the lesions are everywhere, so it is easy to see why there is pain.'

Sophie also has superficial endometriosis and feels that women like her 'tend not to be thought of so much'. She describes herself as 'just someone with lots of pain.'

It can be much more helpful to think about the symptoms than the type of endometriosis when it comes to how women are supported. However, the type of endometriosis is more relevant when it comes to the specific surgical treatment – which we'll explore a bit more in the next chapter.

Diagnostic tests

Pelvic ultrasound and MRI

Endometriosis can only be definitively diagnosed by laparoscopy, so one of the challenges is that tests such as scans, both ultrasound and MRI, don't always show up endometriosis.

While endometriomas, or endometriosis cysts on the ovaries, would normally show up on an ultrasound scan or MRI, endometriosis in other areas does not often show up. But the real challenge can be that a woman with suspected endometriosis might end up having a whole range of other tests – some of them to exclude other diagnoses – and these can be extensive.

Blood tests

While there are no definitive blood tests for endometriosis, a woman with suspected endometriosis may well have not only standard blood tests that look, for example, at white blood cell counts and indicators for inflammation, but may also end up having tests such as a CA125 level. This is a test for a protein in the blood, called 'cancer antigen 125'. It's more commonly used as a test for ovarian cancer but some – not all – women with endometriosis have raised levels of this marker. It is increased with any condition that leads to 'inflammation' in the body, and so it is not helpful on its own as a diagnostic test for endometriosis. Also, a negative test is unable to rule out endometriosis.

Laparoscopy

Endometriosis can only be definitively diagnosed with a laparoscopy. This type of surgery is used to confirm a diagnosis of endometriosis, because the gynaecologist is able to see first-hand the disease and how it has manifested itself. It also gives them the opportunity to 'biopsy' it – to send a sample of it to the lab for analysis, to confirm that it is indeed endometriosis. A laparoscopy may identify signs of previous infection, such as pelvic inflammatory disease or adhesions (scar tissue). Sometimes a woman may be having a laparoscopy for abdominal symptoms where endometriosis is not suspected, so it may be found coincidentally, so there isn't always time to prepare for the diagnosis.

What does a laparoscopy to diagnose endometriosis involve?

Most women are nervous before a laparoscopy – after all, if it's the first time you're either having an operation or a laparoscopy, it's an unknown. It involves having a general anaesthetic and most women will have a 'pre-op' appointment of some sort, where any tests can be done, such as blood tests, heart rate and blood pressure and the procedure can be fully explained. You'll normally be weighed and given any specific instructions for the surgery itself, such as when to stop eating and drinking beforehand. These instructions are vital and must be followed exactly.

On the day, having surgery itself can involve a lot of waiting around – checking in for the surgery itself, meeting doctors involved in your care, such as the anaesthetist, who will explain the procedure and the risks of it, signing consent forms for the operation, waiting your turn on the list and then changing into a gown and surgical stockings for the operation. So, you're now waiting for your first laparoscopy, you're a little nervous, having never done this before. And it's surgery – so it's a big deal to be doing this. But you desperately want and need answers.

An hour or two later after your surgery and you're in the recovery room, phew, hmm this morphine is definitely helping as you come round, things are really fuzzy, you're feeling distinctly woozy and ever-so sleepy, maybe a little nauseous and rather sore but for now you're just going to rest. Ah...

But wait! The gynaecologist is here, they're beside you, they've got a furrowed brow and they're saying something. What are they saying? They found WHAT? Endo something or other? What's that?

You now know it's endometriosis but have no idea what this means

You've entered the third stage – the 'unknown known' – you have a diagnosis but you may have absolutely no idea what it means. Some women have been well prepared before surgery, if endometriosis was suspected. But for others, after surgery might be the first time they hear the word 'endometriosis' and it can be a real shock, particularly when surgeons start talking about highly sensitive issues, like fertility, when a woman is in the recovery room and still coming round from an anaesthetic.

In an ideal world, the immediate aftermath of surgery wouldn't be the time to find out you have the most unpronounceable disease that you've probably ever heard. This may even be the first time you hear the word. But we never promised you an ideal world, we're dealing with reality here. You're one of many patients, your gynaecologist has had a long day in the operating theatre. They may be running behind and they're doing their best.

Providing high-quality information to women with endometriosis is about more than the timing and manner of those explanations, though clearly those matter. From the women we interviewed, what is explained and who delivers this information is also vital.

Let's hear again from women, because whether they were diagnosed last week or ten years ago, they are unlikely to forget the moment they found out their diagnosis. As Lucy explains: 'He woke me up afterwards and he just tapped me on the shoulder and said "I didn't find any adhesions but I did find endometriosis, good luck!" And walked off.'

If you're going to find out that you've got a disease you've never heard of before, the first communication on this is key, Zoe explains: 'To be told by a surgeon when you're 21 that it's unlikely that you'll be able to have children naturally, and fairly bluntly, it sort of sets the tone for the rest of your endo journey.'

And then for others, it can be more dramatic, as Daisy explains: 'I remember coming round from my operation and him standing there and I was on morphine and out of it, and he just said "It's not cancer, it's an endometrioma", and I had literally no idea what he meant.'

Immediately after surgery, and on morphine, is not the time to be asking questions about something you've never heard of, but sadly sometimes this is all the healthcare system allows. However, some women remember their gynaecologist going into a lot of detail, which can be frightening.

> *The doctor wasn't particularly kind in the way he told me about what I had, and he made me feel more scared by what he told me. He told me that it was the worst endometriosis that he'd ever seen, that he wasn't able to treat it, he had no idea how to deal with such a case, I would never have children ... I burst into tears. I felt very bitter that I'd been dropped a bombshell and then left like that without any answers or explanation as to how that would affect me.* – Madison

After surgery, it's worth knowing that your gynaecologist sends a follow-up letter (called a 'discharge letter') to your GP to tell them about your procedure, what was found and what the next steps are. You can ask to be sent a copy of it.

We'll look in more detail at laparoscopic surgery to treat endometriosis in Chapter 2, but here are some hints and tips if you're about to have a laparoscopy:

Hints and tips if you're having a laparoscopy

- Take some time to plan beforehand: this might be, for example, arranging for someone to come and look after you for a few days, buying some new comfy pyjamas, ensuring you have food in the fridge/freezer that is quick and easy to prepare after surgery or making childcare arrangements if required to allow you the time to recover from your surgery.
- Eat a healthy, well-balanced diet in the days running up to your surgery to ensure your bowel is working well. Follow carefully any instructions about when to stop eating and drinking before your operation as this is very important.
- Bring someone with you for support. You won't be able to drive home after surgery and will need someone with you for the first 24 hours after a general anaesthetic.
- Bring loose clothing and comfy underwear to wear afterwards, as well as sanitary towels (not tampons) – your abdomen will be quite swollen from being inflated with air to allow the surgeons to see all around your pelvis during your surgery and there may be some bleeding afterwards.
- Take a small overnight bag – although many laparoscopies are done as day cases, sometimes you can end up staying overnight and it helps to be prepared.

- Remember to bring into hospital any medication that you normally take.
- Bring something to read, some relaxing music to listen to on headphones, or puzzles or any other similar distractions for before the surgery – you may have to wait around before going down to theatre and it helps to have something to do to relax you.
- Before surgery, you will see someone from your surgical team – either your consultant or one of their team – along with the anaesthetist who will explain what will be done – they are there to address any questions or fears you may have, so don't be afraid to ask anything you need to know. Make sure that you know exactly what the surgeon is planning to do. If the endometriosis is superficial you may be asked to consent to having it treated there and then. If it is more complex, ask for the surgery to be carried out at a later date when you have had time to consider the possible consequences of the surgery. Ideally, you only want to have one 'treatment' surgery so it is important that this is carried out by an endometriosis expert and that all of the endometriosis is removed. Write a list of things that you want to ask beforehand and bring this with you as a reminder. Ask your surgeon to take pictures during the surgery – you may see these afterwards – but even if you don't want to see them they can be a very helpful record if you need any further surgery in the future.
- After the laparoscopy, you may experience referred pain in your shoulders (shoulder tip pain) as the gas starts to dissipate – this can be quite painful. Along

with any prescribed pain relief, some women find peppermint oil or peppermint tea helps.

- Having a laparoscopy, like after any general anaesthetic, can sometimes make you feel quite weepy and emotional for a few days afterwards – this is entirely normal and should pass. It is really important to have people around you who are sympathetic, supportive and who understand you might be feeling a bit low.

- You may have two or more small cuts in your abdomen – these may be sealed with surgical glue or stitches, which may be dissolvable or may need to be removed. Your wound sites should be kept covered and dry for a few days after surgery – you should be advised about how to care for them before you are discharged from hospital. If you experience redness, oozing from the wounds or feel unwell, speak to your GP for advice.

- When travelling home after your laparoscopy bring a pillow in the car to hold gently against your abdomen, to help cushion against bumps in the road.

- Constipation can be an issue due to drugs like morphine that may be used during an operation. It's really important to eat a healthy diet, with plenty of fruit and vegetables, after surgery to help avoid constipation. If you have any problems, you could talk to someone from the ward, your pharmacist or GP.

- When it comes to recovery, everyone is different and it will depend on what you had done during the lapa-roscopy. Some women may be back at work within a week or two, some may take longer. The only thing that matters is for you to take whatever time you and your GP or consultant believes is appropriate. Remember, just as your disease is unique to you, so is your treatment and your recovery.

- For advice on when you might be able to drive, resume exercise or have sexual intercourse, always talk to your GP, clinical nurse specialist or consultant. You won't be able to drive for the first 48 hours after a general anaesthetic for insurance purposes and you should not drive until you feel comfortable doing an emergency stop.

- Plan ways to ensure you spend time resting – arrange to have your favourite box sets, DVDs and books close to hand to ensure you take time out to rest.

- Dress in loose and comfortable clothes as you will be bloated after laparoscopic surgery. You won't be able to bend down easily for a few days so you might like to wear slip-on shoes.

- You'll be given advice about bathing and showering by the ward. You may want to have some baby wipes on hand to freshen up.

- If you experience any unusual symptoms after surgery, contact the ward directly or speak to your GP.

Bowel investigations

These may be performed in women with endometriosis who have bowel symptoms. Diarrhoea, constipation, bloating and nausea are common, not just with deep endometriosis that develops on or even in the bowel, but with all types of endometriosis as we don't fully understand it. The investigations can range from sigmoi-doscopies and colonoscopies, where a telescope is used to look inside the bowel, to barium enemas, where a sub-stance that shows up on X-rays is inserted into the bowel to see if there is any structural abnormality, and to other types of X-ray.

Amanda was subsequently diagnosed with deep endometriosis in the bowel. She describes the various tests she had: 'I had enemas and X-rays just to see if anything was going on, and he told me I had a strange-shaped bowel – that was obviously the blockage starting where the endo had infiltrated the bowel. He tried to do a colonoscopy on me and he couldn't even get the paediatric one through because it was so narrow. It was agony.'

Thankfully, sigmoidoscopies and colonoscopies are usually painless and often performed under sedation – you can read more about this test opposite, where we've included hints and tips if you're having a colonoscopy.

It's important to note that for many women, these bowel investigations are being performed prior to diagnosis, meaning that women may be suffering and are desperate for an answer. Bowel investigations can be hard – and performed at a time when you might be quite unwell and without a diagnosis.

If you're going to have a colonoscopy you will probably be feeling a bit nervous, and maybe a little embarrassed. Please be assured that probably everyone who has this done has felt a little unsure about it. Anything to do with the bowel can have us feeling a little alarmed. So, let's have an honest, upfront look at this because it may be on your list of investigations if you're having bowel symptoms related to your endometriosis.

What does it involve?

The first part of the colonoscopy – which is sometimes the part that people fear most – is the cleansing of the intestines so that they are clean so that the doctors performing the colonoscopy (basically a long telescope that goes up your bottom) have a clear view.

This normally involves drinking – over the course of 12 or more hours – a special laxative drink. The hospital or pharmacist provides the instructions for your laxative drink. Note that you should always ask for advice about what to do before your colonoscopy from your consultant, a GP, nurse specialist or pharmacist.

You may plan a little ahead, so the day or two before you take your laxative you could eat a light or 'low-residue' diet, basically a diet that is quite bland and doesn't include much fibre. This includes things like mashed potato, eggs, milk, white fish, chicken and white bread.

When you check the instructions on your laxative, it can sound like a lot to drink. Depending on the bowel preparation that is used, this can be up to a couple of litres. It isn't always the tastiest of drinks so here are a few tips to make it more palatable:

STEP ONE – GET CHILLIN'!

Prepare your drink a little in advance and put it in the fridge; chilling it makes it easier to drink. You may even want to pop some ice into it. It's also easier to drink with a straw.

STEP TWO – WHAT'S YOUR FLAVOUR?

Consider preparing it using one of your favourite cordials. Our top recommendation is ginger cordial but take your pick – in fact, pick a couple so you can have a selection and vary it a bit. You might fancy a different flavour for the second serving, if your drink requires it. Add the cordial when you are ready to drink.

STEP THREE – GET COMFY AT HOME!

Consider how you are going to while away the time whilst you drink the laxative. Perhaps watching the latest box set or movie, or listening to your favourite music. Whatever you plan to do, ensure you have a comfy place to relax in reasonably close proximity to the loo. Stock up on wet wipes, loo roll and nappy rash cream as you may get a bit sore after the bowel movements.

How long does it take?

The laxative may start to work before you finish the first round of drinks. Not everyone finds it works as quickly, again we are all different. However, as the hours progress, your bowel will gradually, or maybe even quite rapidly, be emptied.

You won't be able to eat until after the actual colonoscopy, as the bowel needs to be completely empty.

Part two – the colonoscopy

Feeling rather empty and quite a bit slimmer, you head off to the hospital for your colonoscopy. This is the time for your partner, family member or friend to drive you to and from wherever you need to be, as most colonoscopies are performed under sedation and you won't be able to drive for 24 hours afterwards.

THE JOURNEY DOWN UNDER . . . .

This is the part we can't tell you much about. Five seconds of thinking – that telescope thingy is going to go into your bottom and suddenly the gin and tonic feeling of sedation hits, then you're asleep ... then you're waking up in recovery. It's all over. You remember nothing. Ah. Partly you are sorry not to have watched the screen for that journey into the depths of your large intestine, partly you are just so relieved it's over. Afterwards, you might feel a little tired and windy for a while. It's important to take it easy for the rest of the day and be kind to yourself.

But what may they have found? A colonoscopy may be used as much to exclude diagnoses that affect the bowel (such as inflammatory bowel diseases) when a woman is experiencing bowel symptoms. It would rarely be used to diagnose endometriosis – but it is a common procedure to investigate persistent bowel symptoms.

Urological investigations

These are less common, probably because endometriosis of the urological tract—that is the bladder, ureters and kidneys—is less common. However, even in cases where endometriosis is not identified either on or in the bladder, it can cause bladder symptoms such as pain and frequency of passing urine. This is also not fully understood, but it can mean that women end up undergoing tests on this area of the body.

> *I had repeated renal IVUs and CT contrast scans. I had bladder capacity scans and CTs of my abdomen. I'd had repeated ultrasounds, internal and external. I had lots of blood tests, smears, lots of repeated investigations, internally, vaginally and rectally.* – Sophie

In rare cases, endometriosis can block the ureter and urine exiting the kidney, causing the kidney to enlarge (hydronephrosis) and become painful. It is important that this is diagnosed early as it can cause long-term kidney damage if left untreated. An ultrasound or MRI that focuses on the renal tract, or CT intravenous urogram (CT IVU) that uses contrast material injected into veins, will detect hydronephrosis.

These are a lot of tests to be subjected to – and that is the point. You might have a negative ultrasound test, or even an MRI, but you could end up having a whole array of tests and investigations. This is as much a process of exclusion as inclusion but it can be exhausting and upsetting to undergo all these procedures.

Even with the most advanced scans, there are limitations, and it can be hard to pick up a full picture of the disease. Consultant gynaecologist Andrew Kent describes firstly how he relies on taking an accurate history from the woman. 'If I have a patient who has come to see me with pelvic pain, I will take a detailed history with specific questions about endometriosis and the pain itself. What you are trying to do, in asking these questions, is to ascertain the nature of the pain to give an idea of whether it could be superficial or deep endometriosis or something else. The examination is tailored to confirm or refute the conclusions that you have come to in your patient's history and allows you to draw up a list of differential diagnoses. A scan is not always required at this stage.'

Ultimately, he explains, only seeing it and feeling the areas of disease through a laparoscopy gives the surgeon all the information that they need to make an assessment about the overall treatment plan. 'Even with the most detailed scans, you cannot get all the information required to allow a clear treatment plan. You can pick up endometriomas easily with ultrasound and MRI, but even an MRI does not provide you with all the information needed to plan surgery, especially with the more severe forms of the disease.'

Myths about endometriosis

If the absence of information and the delivery of a diagnosis of endometriosis is challenging for a woman, it can be even harder to then have to deal with some of the reactions from doctors, family, friends or colleagues, however well-meaning. It's great when people have actually heard of endometriosis, but it can be equally frustrating dealing with some of the myths about it.

Often this involves women with endometriosis having to explain to others about what is really going on. Since this is a disease that affects everyone very differently, adopting an open and honest attitude to people's comments can help to clear up any misunderstandings, however frustrating they are.

We've already looked at 'normal pain' – what it means to be a woman who suffers with painful periods and knowing what is 'normal' – as well as some of the myths that surround that. We've seen how this impacts on the journey to obtain a diagnosis for endometriosis. Sadly, some of the most common myths relate to things that 'cure' endometriosis. We should add at this stage that the notion of 'curing' endometriosis is quite controversial, but more of this later.

Myth #1 'I know someone who had endometriosis and she's cured now'

Sadly, although many women have successful treatment for endometriosis, there is, as yet, no known 'cure'. Of course, there are many women who feel a lot better after treatment, but this isn't going to help the woman on the receiving end of this statement to manage her symptoms and handle all that goes with endometriosis.

Friends, family and colleagues should adopt a listening, supportive approach – offering empathy and comfort. The experience of others is very unlikely to help a woman at this point in time, however listening to her explain her individual circumstances and challenges is likely to be beneficial to everyone. Asking open-ended questions, showing genuine interest and not jumping to offer solutions – these are excellent ways to approach women with endometriosis.

They think you can just take the tablets and it's curable, and it's not like that, so I think, if I'm explicit then he knows he can ask questions. – Lucy, talking about her colleague

Myth #2 'Have a baby, you'll be cured'

This is probably one of the most upsetting things a woman with endometriosis can hear. First of all, it is wholly inappropriate to suggest pregnancy to a woman as a cure for a gynaecological disease. Some women may be desperately struggling to get pregnant – it is estimated that around a third of infertile women seeking fertility treatment have endometriosis and some are only diagnosed as part of this process. Secondly, whilst some – but not all – women experience a reduction in pain through pregnancy and whilst breastfeeding, they may well experience a return of pain and resurgence of the disease once their periods restart.

Some women reported that this comment may come from family, friends and even healthcare practitioners.

We'll hear more from women about pregnancy in Chapter 5 and what it really means to be a woman with endometriosis, both during and after pregnancy.

Myth #3 'Have a hysterectomy, you'll be cured'

This is the opposite of the baby myth, but is equally insensitive. Yes, having a hysterectomy stops periods but this is very unlikely to be appropriate as a first-line treatment in a young woman – and it may only be relevant if endometrial-like cells are specifically affecting a woman within the muscular wall of her uterus or womb – a condition called adenomyosis, which you can read more about later in this chapter. If you have a hysterectomy but not all endometriosis is removed at the same time, you may still experience the symptoms of endometriosis.

Luckily, many women have seen a change in this stance in recent years as Nicole notes:

'When I was 21, the first thing my consultant said was you can have a hysterectomy. When I saw him after a few years, he told me that, "No, hysterectomy is a last resort because we've been finding that women have had hysterectomies, the endometriosis is still there, because there were patches of it where we weren't expecting it", so now they will only do it as a last resort unless the woman has particularly asked for it.'

Myth #4 Ethnicity affects your risk of endometriosis

Endometriosis does not affect any one ethnic group more than any other, but we should recognise the importance of racial and cultural differences that may affect attitudes towards pain and fertility, because awareness among some BAME (black and minority ethnic) groups can be lower. Women also reported that sometimes there are damaging stereotypes about different ethnicities and pain thresholds.

'There are many cultural and social norm factors attributable to the higher level of lack of awareness,' Afuah tells us. 'For example, some BAME women don't like to talk about menstruation, especially in public, to the point that if a woman has their period, the men in the household are not told, even when the woman is suffering pain – the general response is "she is not feeling well".'

Endometriosis does indeed not have any barriers – women of any race can be affected – but there may be cultural barriers that deter women from seeking help. It's important to be aware of these. For example, there may be additional pressure to be silent about menstrual problems, and there may also be family pressures to have children. 'It is a less talked-about condition,' explains Sanjeev, whose wife has endometriosis. 'I am the only one who knows about it, about her problem.'

If menstruation is already taboo, raising awareness about endometriosis can be hard, but it needs to be done. Afuah tells us about a woman she has recently worked with. Afuah explains, 'She encouraged her sister, who had unfortunately undergone FGM (female genital mutilation) during childhood, to seek gynaecological help. Previously, all her sister's gynaecological problems were assumed to be due to the FGM. In short, her sister was eventually diagnosed with endometriosis.' Information and education have important roles in this area.

The lowdown on adenomyosis

Adenomyosis is defined by the finding of endometrial-like tissue within the muscular wall of the womb, called the myometrium. The cause of it is not known. It can be difficult to diagnose, but increasingly transvaginal ultrasound and magnetic resonance imaging (MRI) are being used. With transvaginal ultrasound, considerable training is needed to recognise the ultrasound pattern of adenomyosis. With MRI, the findings are less dependent on the person doing the scan, but it still depends on an observer who is expert in reporting such scans in gynaecology. Adenomyosis can be easily confused with fibroids (tumour-like overgrowths of smooth muscle in the uterus that are also associated with heavy periods) on ultrasound and MRI. But, a definitive diagnosis of adenomyosis can only be made with a biopsy (sample of tissue) and histological analysis (examination of the tissue with a microscope in the laboratory). This is not commonly performed for the diagnosis of adenomyosis and so the diagnosis is only usually made after hysterectomy (when the womb is routinely looked at in the laboratory).

Even when a woman has suspected adenomyosis, a hysterectomy is a life-changing operation and whether this is something a woman wishes to consider will depend entirely on her individual circumstances and her personal choice.

Information on the internet

Let's take a look now at one of the most used sources on information about endometriosis, its causes, symptoms and treatments – the internet.

Since many people only hear the word 'endometriosis' when either they themselves are diagnosed with it, or their partner, family member or friend receives a diagnosis, this may often be followed by a scrabble around on the internet to find out a bit more. This can be helpful, but it can also lead to much confusion, because endometriosis is quite an individual disease, not only in the way it presents, but also in how it affects women on a day-to-day basis. One woman's endometriosis is definitely not the same as another's – and so care is definitely required when looking at information on the internet.

There is, however, no doubt that the internet has raised some much-needed awareness about endometriosis – whether that is through social media, celebrities more willingly sharing information about their endometriosis, or the ability to search and access a much wider range of information. The internet has been a very important tool for the sharing of information. This is not just the case for endometriosis – it applies to a wide range of medical conditions or situations. Quite simply, when using the internet, we need to apply two very important human codes: those of common sense and courtesy.

Hints and tips for a positive internet experience

- If looking for general information on a medical condition, always use a reliable source such as a national registered charity or the NHS (including their recommended links).
- The internet is never a place for individual medical opinions – if you have concerns and questions, remember that the best place for these is with your healthcare professional, whether that is your GP, specialist nurse or consultant. They may not have all the answers straightaway but appropriate face-to-face

dialogue with the people who know you and your body is essential. The internet is not the place to do this.

- Social media, blogs, vlogs and chat forums can be invaluable sources of support, where you can meet other people with the same condition and share the challenges, tips and lots of empathy – but their situation may well be very different to your own. Always treat others with respect, in the way that you would wish to be dealt with, and report any concerns to moderators on chat forums. Avoid using personally identifiable information. Be very cautious when applying the experiences of others to your own situation. We are all unique after all, and your endometriosis, like many diseases, is very specific to you.

- Remember the limitations of the internet – you may find the support of others online really useful but there are other ways of receiving support, such as in support groups, contacting charity helplines or through local counselling services. Receiving support or having contact face-to-face or by phone can be enormously beneficial.

- It's worth bearing in mind that women who have mild symptoms or a smooth journey are less likely to report their journey on the internet. There is enough to deal with as a woman with endometriosis, or as a partner to a woman with endo, without adding extra fear – so when it comes to the internet and endometriosis, proceed with caution, common sense and courtesy.

What did the women we interviewed say about the internet?

Women identified both the benefits and drawbacks of the internet. Firstly, it was identified as an important way that family and friends could help them, particularly when newly diagnosed. Sophie really appreciated her dad and boyfriend doing this:

'That evening my boyfriend came home with tons of information printed off the Endometriosis UK website. My dad had done the same. I couldn't believe these two men were researching period stuff and helping me in my darkest hour.... Those actions meant so much.'

But proceed with caution – this isn't everybody's way of working, as Scarlett explained:

'I remember my friend was googling endometriosis because she's a librarian but I said, I don't want you to tell me what it says, I want to find it all out for myself.'

Daisy thinks that social media has led younger women to be more assertive, to take action and to ask for help – which may, in turn, lead to a quicker diagnosis than the seven to eight years it takes, on average, to receive a diagnosis of endometriosis: 'I think we're lucky with the Internet and Facebook. I think the younger girls definitely seem to be thinking to themselves as soon as they hear about it, right, well, what's this, what am I going to do about it? Who's there to help me? And I think that's really brilliant.'

Poppy echoes the concerns about advice given on social-media sites – it's important to distinguish between internet chat and the important medical advice given to us by doctors and nurses: 'I think social media is a really bad thing at times, because it erodes the trust between a woman and her consultant. Sometimes it can be good because you can hear more things and it can actually make you more empowered and more informed, so you can make a more informed choice, but there are too many people out there who are willing to give medical advice when they've got none to give.'

A pain and symptoms diary

Week beginning DD/ MM /YY	Are you on your period?	Describe your pain* and where it is	How does it feel and how long does it last? e.g. 3 hours	Do you have any other symptoms? e.g. bloating, bleeding, bowel or urinary problems	Did you take or do anything to help with the pain or symptoms? If so, what did it help?	What affect did it have on you?**
Mon						
Tues						
Wed						
Thurs						
Fri						
Sat						
Sun						

* Please rate your pain on a scale of 1-10. Where 1 =tolerable and 10 =the worst pain imaginable

** Please state whether these symptoms affected your work, education, relationships, social activities, sleep, exercise, food intake, sex life, stress levels, quality of life that day

Chapter 2

Making choices: treatment options

The diagnosis journey in chapter 1 was quite challenging, wasn't it? You're probably thinking that the treatment of endometriosis should surely be more straightforward, shouldn't it?

Well, this is a disease that doesn't always play by the rules. If diagnosis was frustrating, choosing treatments is very much about selecting a route, trying it out and then choosing plan B if the first route doesn't work out. We can think of it as a bit like satellite navigation, or GPS – we plan a route, but then traffic comes along, or a road gets closed, so we have to divert off and take an altered course. Let's take a closer look at what this really means.

Route planning

We've established a few essential aspects of endometriosis, notably that:

- We don't definitively know what causes it, although it is an inflammatory disease that has an important hormonal element to it.

- Symptoms can be varied but predominantly involve a woman's pelvic organs.

- All women are different in how endometriosis affects them.

- It sometimes takes a long time to diagnose.

So, we just then need to factor in to the 'route planning':

- What a woman's priorities are – is it symptom relief, fertility, or both?

- What previous treatments (including surgery) have been tried, and very importantly, what are her preferences?

Putting all that together sounds quite complex, doesn't it? Well, it is. And on top of that, we can throw into the mix the fact that there are very few drugs that are specifically licensed for the treatment of endometriosis, and this in itself is a huge stumbling block.

Pain medications

The first form of treatment that many women will receive will be in the form of pain medication. There is a wide range of medication available to help control pain. Some of these are available over the counter and are used regularly for conditions like endometriosis, and others are prescription only and are generally taken for shorter periods of time.

Pain medications are an important aspect of pain management for many women with endometriosis, however, there are significant side – effects with some of them. For example, opioids can cause drowsiness and, in long-term use addiction, whereas NSAIDs (see below) can damage the stomach lining.

- Paracetamol is a commonly used over-the-counter medication used to treat fever and mild – to moderate pain.

- Anti-inflammatories, such as ibuprofen or mefenamic acid, are generally referred to as 'NSAIDS' or non-steroidal anti-inflammatories. They are available over the counter or on prescription and are an important group of drugs used to treat endometriosis-related pain. They can cause stomach ulcers and, if taken for any period of time, should be taken with another medication to protect the stomach lining. You should discuss this with your GP.

- Weak opioids such as dihydrocodeine are generally available only on prescription, although weaker forms are available over the counter in combination with paracetamol (e.g. co-codamol). These are used to treat moderate pain and can have side effects such as constipation and dependency

- Stronger opioids such as tramadol, oramorph and morphine are only available on prescription. Side effects of these include sedation, dizziness, nausea, vomiting, constipation, physical dependence, tolerance and respiratory depression. There is a considerable risk of addiction with this type of drug, however, they are normally used short term only, such as after surgery, or whilst awaiting medical or surgical treatment.

- Neuromodulators such as amitriptyline, nortriptyline, duloxetine, gabapentin and pregabalin, are drugs that are used to treat 'neuropathic', or nerve, pain. They are thought to work by altering the functioning of brain regions that are controlled by chemicals in the brain called 'neurotransmitters', which are responsible for transferring messages between brain cells. There is evidence to suggest that they are beneficial for other chronic pain conditions so it is thought that they might help reduce endometriosis pain. They can be taken longer term and are generally increased or decreased slowly. They can cause drowsiness, confusion, blurred vision, weight gain and other side effects. They are only available on prescription and are often used in pain clinics, or when other forms of treatment have failed to provide adequate symptom control. Some neuromodulators are also used as antidepressants (amitriptyline, nortriptyline, duloxetine) but it is important to note that, if they are prescribed for endometriosis, they are usually being used primarily for their pain-relieving qualities.

It's important to discuss your pain with the GP as some women find referral to pain clinics and access to pain psychology services really helpful. We'll look at these in Chapter 3.

Hormone treatments

In general, women will start out on the lower dose hormonal treatments before embarking on more 'heavy-duty' treatments. In fact, nearly all the women we interviewed had already tried one treatment long before they had even been diagnosed with endometriosis: the combined contraceptive pill (COCP). That's a mix of female hormones both released by the ovaries – oestrogen, which is the main female sex hormone, combined with progestin. The two hormones 'trick' the woman's body into believing she is pregnant by stopping the ovaries from releasing an egg every month – this is called 'anovulation'.

So why is this relevant to women with endometriosis? Well, whilst a woman is on the combined pill, her periods are likely to be lighter and less painful (and the pill can even lessen the pain she may experience outside her periods) so although it is licensed as a contraceptive – i.e., to stop a sexually active woman becoming pregnant – it is also used to improve the symptoms of endometriosis.

It can be effective for some, but it is not without issues, and some women experience side effects.

The combined oral contraceptive pill

Many women take the combined pill as teenagers before they receive a diagnosis, taking it for three weeks of the month and having a one-week break where they may have a lighter bleed than a normal period.

Nicole started taking the pill when painkillers weren't working as well as previously. 'My mum took me to the doctors, they gave me mefenamic acid and ibuprofen and just said "oh get on with it", you know, "this is your life, this is what being a woman is like", so I carried on until I was about 16 and then they said "okay, we'll try the pill", so they put me on the pill and it was all right. I'd get three weeks of okay and then a week where obviously I took a break because they didn't really know it was endometriosis.'

Sophie also waited until she was 16 to start taking the pill and found it really helped her symptoms at this point: 'I regularly saw the GP who wanted to start me on the pill but my mum was not keen on this so I didn't go on it until I was 16. At this point, it really helped with my periods and helped to make them a lot lighter.'

Not all women found the pill helped when they were teenagers. Saskia was one of these girls: 'I went on the pill for a little while when I was about 13, 14 maybe, and the GP said: "well, periods do hurt and there can be a bit of pain, but maybe you can try going on the pill for a little while and see if that helps", and it didn't really but nobody said it was a big deal and as a teenager you trust what your parents are saying and what the doctors are saying.'

Amanda went to her doctor with heavy, painful periods in her teens and was given the pill. She tells us that it was effective, but her symptoms returned as soon as she came off it. 'When I got married, when I decided to come off the pill because it wasn't a problem if I fell pregnant, I had awful pains, I'd pass out, doubled-over every period.'

Whilst women either got some, or a lot of relief from the pill when they were suffering as teenagers, they consistently reported that their symptoms came back once they stopped, with many women referring to the way the pill had 'masked' their disease. It is in looking back that perhaps women felt they did not have the complete picture, because they did not have a diagnosis.

The contraceptive pill still is an important and effective treatment for heavy, painful periods and, whilst we await a better diagnostic tool, we can expect that women with symptoms will continue to be prescribed this treatment, but we can hope that communication between women and doctors about endometriosis may improve, so that women receive a possible diagnosis for their symptoms, and coming off the pill and the symptoms returning is not a surprise.

So, if coming off the pill may be a problem, surely one solution is to go back on it? Well, it's not quite that simple and there are many reasons why a woman may want to – or have to – stop taking the pill, including trying to get pregnant.

It's worth also considering that when the pill is prescribed to women with a diagnosis of endometriosis, it may be taken in a slightly different way than when taken as a contraceptive. Why is this?

Gynaecologists who prescribe the pill to women with endometriosis may prescribe it to be taken 'back to back'. What that means is that instead of having three weeks on and then a break for a week to have a light bleed, women may take it without any break at all, perhaps for a period of three months or longer ('tri-cycling'), when they then have a short break to have a bleed. In this way, periods are minimised and therefore the bleeding from endometriosis lesions is also minimised.

Thea started taking the pill in this way following major surgery for bowel endometriosis. She started by tri-cycling the pill, taking it for three months and then having a short break, but then started taking it continuously: 'I take the combined pill now and it was my consultant who put me on that. I was originally on it on a tri-cycle basis but then when I saw him in the follow-up appointment he said that I could take it continuously. He said to me there was no reason why you can't, he basically said it's better for me the fewer cycles I have, the less chance of it reoccurring.' So, we've seen that the pill may have a role to play to help women, but what can women do if this route is not working or is not a viable option, perhaps due to the side – effects a woman experiences?

Progesterone-based treatments

At this stage, one of the questions you might have is this: if endometriosis is a disease that depends on hormones – and in particular oestrogen, the main female sex hormone – why would a treatment that combines both oestrogen and progestin, the synthetic form of progesterone, be used to treat symptoms of endometriosis?

Well, this is a difficult and interesting question. Progestogens (the term that describes the body's natural progesterone and synthetic progestins) are thought to work by stimulating 'atrophy' or regression – wasting away – of endometrial lesions. But their effectiveness in treating endometriosis is not just linked to their 'growth inhibiting' actions, but linked to the fact that they can cause anovulation. This is when the ovaries do not release an oocyte (a cell that forms an egg) during the menstrual cycle). They also result in lower oestrogen levels, slow down blood vessel growth, and are anti-inflammatory.

Some women may find that using a progestin-only treatment is beneficial for relieving symptoms. These can be prescribed in several different ways, including the mini pill and within an implant placed inside the uterus, called the Mirena™ coil (or intra-uterine system, IUS), which releases small amounts of progestin and lasts for up to five years. The mini pill involves a higher dose of progestin but has the advantage of flexibility – you can stop it whenever you like – whereas the Mirena™ uses significantly smaller amounts of the drug because it is situated inside the uterus and therefore less drug is needed. The Mirena™ needs to be inserted by a trained healthcare professional and must also be removed by one – it's not a short-term treatment so it does need to fit in with a woman's long-term plans.

Other progestogen treatments include the long-acting progestin injection (such as Depo-Provera™), which is given into the muscle or under the skin every eight or twelve weeks; a progestin implant that is put under the skin in order to offer you an even dose that lasts up to three years (such as Nexplanon™); and a tablet called Norethisterone, which is another synthetic progestin that is taken daily. Essentially, these all have similar effects of reducing the bleeding a woman experiences and therefore minimising bleeding from endometriosis lesions.

What did women tell us about progestogen-only treatments? Experiences were divided – but again we should remind you that every woman responds differently.

Norethisterone

Madison has been taking Norethisterone for some years, which is not specifically licensed to be taken for endometriosis in this way but it suits her well: 'After the bowel surgery I've been put onto a medication where I have a very low dose of a drug that stops my periods so I don't ovulate at all, so since my surgery I have managed to maintain this very low dosage. I've had a great recovery from the surgery and I've managed to stay very well in terms of endometriosis. I recently had a scan and I don't actually have any endometriosis showing at all and I haven't had any recurrence of endometriomas.'

Mirena™ coil

Some women experience excellent symptom relief from the Mirena™, which can last for up to five years before it needs to be replaced.

Afuah had her Mirena™ coil inserted after many years of endometriosis, including several laparoscopies and two pregnancies. She has experienced long-term symptom relief. 'Currently, my endometriosis symptoms are well controlled with the Mirena™ coil, which I call "my second friend" because it's been amazing. I have been quite stable on it. I have been symptom-free on it since then and I have just had it replaced.'

However, five years of symptom relief is certainly not guaranteed. 'I had a Mirena™ coil inserted,' Lucy tells us, 'and then I was fine for two years.' After this time Lucy found her symptoms started to return.

Some women find that symptoms will be improved rather than eliminated as Emily found: 'I've got the Mirena™, it's settled really well for me. It doesn't solve things but it's definitely an improvement.'

A Mirena™ coil may be inserted by your gynaecologist, GP or in a family planning or sexual health clinic. Some women may be anxious about having the coil inserted or removed and replaced. It can sometimes be more painful and potentially harder to insert when women have not had children. Some hospital centres that treat women with endometriosis may insert coils under sedation, or sometimes they are inserted at the same time as a laparoscopy when a woman is under a general anaesthetic.

There can be challenges with the Mirena™ coil. It's not for everybody and it can take a few months to settle, in which time a woman may have to cope with erratic bleeding, which can be troublesome. That said, for some, persistence pays off and things settle down.

Poppy still has bleeding with her coil, and wonders what is happening inside. 'Although I'm on the Mirena™ now, and I have been for over a year, I still do get a bleed; it's not every month but I still do get a bleed.'

If the Mirena™ can sometimes be challenging to insert, removal is generally much easier and can often be done by GPs who have trained to do this. The Mirena™ can be a great option for some women but it is not suitable for everyone. Why is this?

Scarlett's gynaecologist was simply unable to put the Mirena™ coil inside her because her endometriosis was so severe at that stage. 'I woke up from the surgery and he said to me, "oh there's been a complication, I couldn't get the coil in".' Scarlett later went on to have a hysterectomy and bowel surgery for severe endometriosis.

So, there may be times when the coil simply cannot be fitted. We also cannot ignore the fact that some women dislike the idea of having an object inserted into an area of the body that is already painful.

The Mirena™ coil, like all the other progestogen treatments mentioned, was developed as a contraceptive and is not specifically licensed for the treatment of endometriosis, however it remains an important treatment option for women with endometriosis. But it isn't a solution for everyone. So, what other treatment routes are available?

Other hormone-like treatments

As you can imagine, with a disease like endometriosis it often isn't a question of having one surgery or one course of treatment and then the job is done – sometimes that is the case, which is wonderful. But for many women, the journey may well involve several different treatments or surgeries – or sometimes even many of them. What happens when we hit a roadblock, or have to take a detour on this long journey?

At this point, the treatments start to get a lot more intense. We're talking about higher doses of hormones, ones that trick women's bodies into thinking they're in the menopause. And that's a very serious thought, especially for a young woman.

Why would women consider these drugs? Well, firstly the simpler contraceptive-type treatments don't work for everyone, or perhaps some women don't achieve long-term symptom relief from them. Secondly, there may be specific times, such as before certain types of surgery, where these drugs are used to dampen down the disease to make the process of surgery more straightforward.

GnRH agonists

So what are these treatments and how do they work? These treatments are called gonadotropin releasing hormone agonists, or GnRH agonists, and they work by reducing the body's production of oestrogen and testosterone – you may think of this as the 'male hormone' but it is also found in lower levels in women. That's why they're not only used for endometriosis, but they're also an important part of treating certain hormone-dependent cancers, such as prostate cancer in men and certain breast cancers in women. Some of the drugs used are:

- Goserelin, known by the brand name Zoladex™.

- Triptorelin, known by the brand name Decapeptyl™.

- Leuprorelin, known by the brand names Prostap™ or Lupron™.

There are also others that may be used, e.g. Buserelin and Naferelin, that are delivered by nasal spray.

These drugs work by blocking oestrogen and progesterone production, so the woman is put straight into a temporary menopausal state, her periods cease, and therefore the endometriosis lesions are thought to become less 'active'. Drugs can be given via an injectable implant either on a monthly, or even three-monthly basis. Once the injection has been delivered, the drug takes effect quickly, but once the month or three months is up, the drug either needs to be re-administered or the effects are reversed. That means not only that the woman will come out of her temporary menopause, but also that any remaining endometriosis will again become active – unless it is removed by surgery at this stage.

These drugs are licensed for six months for the treatment of endometriosis and the three-monthly preparation is not licensed for endometriosis at all, but they can be given for longer or as the three-monthly preparation if a woman wishes. Why are they licensed for only six months? Well, although the effects of the temporary menopause are reversible, these are 'heavy-duty' hormones with significant side effects (such as thinning of the bones – increasing the risk of osteoporosis). It is recommended that if women use GnRH analogues beyond six months, that they also take 'add-back HRT' with them; that's using traditional hormone replacement therapy combining small amounts of oestrogen and progestin to help relieve some of the menopause symptoms and side effects.

As we take another pitstop to hear again from women on their experiences of these drugs, it is worth again considering that these medications form the main body of drugs currently licensed for the treatment of endometriosis – and yet they are only licensed for six months. This is obviously sadly at odds with a disease that can potentially affect a woman for the whole of her reproductive life and occasionally beyond that.

Women told us that, when it came to GnRH agonists, they often experienced a lot of relief from their endometriosis symptoms. Sophie says: 'Zoladex totally gave me my life back, I managed to get back to work on it.'

Sophie wasn't able to have add-back HRT throughout her treatment due to a family history of breast cancer and cardiac problems. Some women did take add-back HRT with their GnRH drugs, as Olivia did. She tells us her consultant 'suggested I try Prostap again but with HRT, so I tried that, and actually it gave me a new lease of life for, I'd say about 12 months.'

A few women had taken GnRH agonists prior to major bowel surgery for endometriosis, women like Thea, who says, 'He then started me on Zoladex before I had the op. It was about six months, because not only have they got to find the time for those two surgeons to be free together, but he wanted to give it a good amount of time for the Zoladex to kick in, for the inflammation to go down and hopefully make the surgery a bit easier once they're in.'

Madison also had GnRH treatment before bowel surgery and felt that whilst she had some side effects, the benefits outweighed these. 'I don't think it was as bad as I was expecting it to be, I mean the hot flushes weren't brilliant; I got hot at night, but actually the fact that it stops your periods, I didn't feel overly emotional on it, so I really didn't find Zoladex that bad at all. And it obviously did the job for quietening down everything for the next operation.'

But does it work for everyone? No, it doesn't, unfortunately – but then there isn't one single treatment that works for all women, so this is no surprise. For some women, the range of side effects outweighed any improvements to their symptoms. Zoe told us, 'I tried Zoladex, which was a pretty horrific six months. It didn't really alleviate the pain, it induced menopause, and even with HRT, I just felt so unwell for that period of time.'

Sometimes women may be offered these heavy-duty hormones at a time when perhaps they have not had chance to ask questions, or the effects of it have not been fully explained to them. This occasionally means that women believe they have been given a treatment that would cure them completely. Olivia explains, 'So for me, I thought it's like having an infection where you have antibiotics, you've just got to do this for a certain while and then you'll be fine at the end of it, so I was quite happy with that and thought oh, fair enough if it's helps. The Zoladex didn't really improve things for me.'

Chloe took GnRH agonists with add-back HRT and weighed the side effects she experienced, such as hot flushes, hair loss and restless legs against the benefits she obtained. Chloe was able to rediscover the woman that she was without endometriosis. 'The exercise that I do now, there is no way I would have even contemplated cycling to the end of the road, let alone doing 120 miles or whatever … for everything that you lose with the injection, you can gain so much because it gives you and your system the opportunity to see what life could be like. And even if there are some side effects, they aren't going to be there for ever.'

In short, these treatments can be tough – the side effects individually, the appropriateness of taking HRT as an add-back therapy and the impact of the treatment on a woman are very personal – but these drugs mean that sometimes women return to work, or are able to resume important hobbies and interests, to do the things that make them happy. We leave the final comments on these drugs to Chloe, whose life has been heavily impacted by deep endometriosis:

You talk to the doctors and the doctors are saying, it's all right, all it's doing is switching off the signal between your brain and your womb. But your womb and your ovaries are vital organs, so, you know, that's like a mainframe of what keeps your body going. So as much as it was sabotaging my body, it was also doing a really vital job. So going on Zoladex for me, I think for any woman, is a big deal.—Chloe

Aromatase inhibitors

Rarely, 'aromatase inhibitors' are prescribed for women with endometriosis who have not had success with other treatments or who cannot use them because of their side effects. Aromatase is a protein in the body that is responsible for producing oestrogen. Normally, it is found in the ovaries, and to a much lesser extent in the skin and fat.

Research has shown that aromatase is also found in high levels in the lesions of women with endometriosis, and that inhibiting the aromatase by giving women an aromatase inhibitor suppresses the growth of their endometriosis, and reduces the associated inflammation. The aromatase inhibitors used for endometriosis include letrozole and anastrozole.

To date, only a few studies involving a limited number of women have been carried out, but these studies indicate that aromatase inhibitors markedly reduce the amount of endometriosis and pelvic pain in most women. These drugs are used to treat some breast cancers but they are still in the experimental phase for treatment of endometriosis, and it will take more research to see if, in the longer term, they provide an effective treatment. Like all the hormonal treatments for endometriosis, aromatase inhibitors will not improve a woman's chance of conceiving, so they should not be used as a treatment for infertility.

Hormone treatments: a summary

We've looked in detail at a lot of different hormonal medication, so let's take a look at this in summary:

Treatment	What is it?	How long can I take it for?*	Pros	Cons
Combined oral contraceptive pill (oestrogen and progestin)	Pill, taken daily for 21 days with a seven-day break (can be taken continuously e.g. 'tri-cycling')	Years	Convenient and easy to take Can be prescribed and monitored by a GP Effects can be stopped quickly if required Method of birth control	Side effects in some women Can't be taken when trying to get pregnant
Mini pill (progestin only)	Pill, taken daily	Years	Convenient and easy to take Can be prescribed and monitored by a GP Effects can be stopped quickly if required Method of birth control	Side effects in some women Can't be taken when trying to get pregnant
Norethisterone	Pill, taken daily	Generally up to six months but can be taken for longer	Convenient and easy to take Can be prescribed and monitored by a GP Effects can be stopped quickly if required	Side effects in some women Can't be taken when trying to get pregnant
Mirena™ coil	Implant inserted into uterus containing progestin	Years (one implant lasts up to five years)	A lower dose of progestin than pills Can be very effective for some women	Requires insertion and removal by a clinician Insertion can be painful May take months to settle down and cause pain and bleeding during this time

Depo-Provera™	Injection, every three months	Years	Needs visits to doctor every 12 weeks Can cause loss of bone density and other side effects
GnRH agonist	Injection every month or every three months OR Nasal spray	Six months (but can be prescribed by a gynaecologist for longer with appropriate monitoring) * Refers to licensed period of time. In practice, some women may use some drugs for longer periods. Consult your doctor for advice.	Can be an effective treatment in some 'Add back' HRT reduces menopausal side effects and loss of bone density	Menopausal side effects, which can be severe in some Causes loss of bone density
Aromatase inhibitors	Pill, taken daily	No current recommended guidance	Not a widely used treatment currently	Menopausal side effects, which can be severe in some Causes loss of bone density

Surgery

Surgery is a large topic and can be a really important route not only to definitively diagnose endometriosis, but also to manage the disease and its symptoms. The aim of surgery when used as a 'treatment' is to completely remove or 'destroy' the endometriosis.

Endometriosis surgery, as you can probably imagine, ranges from straightforward to highly complex gynaecological procedures that involve a range of other surgeons and specialities, such as colorectal and urology. Most surgeries for endometriosis are done using a laparoscopic (keyhole) approach. Here, we discuss the role of surgery for endometriosis in general, with a focus on surgery to treat pain, and in Chapter 5, we look specifically at endometriosis surgery for infertility.

Laparoscopic surgery to treat endometriosis

Laparoscopic surgery for endometriosis always involves a general anaesthetic, so you're asleep for the operation. It involves making two or more small cuts on the abdomen, usually in the belly button and then others surrounding that, depending on what is to be done. These cuts are about 5–10mm each and are often referred to by the medical team as 'port sites' because they will be used to hold a specific instrument – firstly, the laparoscope, which is a short instrument with a camera on the end that the surgeon uses to see what is going on, and secondly a tube that pumps carbon dioxide gas into the abdomen, so it's inflated to allow room for the surgeons to do their work. There may be up to five or six ports for more complex surgery as many different instruments may be used to move, cut or burn diseased tissue, depending on what is being done. The images from the laparoscope are shown on a large screen and are highly magnified, so everyone in the operating theatre has a really good view of what is going on.

Who's in the operating theatre? Well, apart from the gynaecologist, there will be the anaesthetist and then a selection of other staff including several scrub nurses, who look after all the instruments, various staff assisting the gynaecologist such as more junior doctors who are specialising in the field and training, as well as doctors assisting the anaesthetist. Everyone is there to make sure the operation goes as smoothly as possible and that the woman is treated with the best possible care before, during and after surgery. Even before a woman is anaesthetised, various observations are made, such as blood pressure and heart rate, and from the moment the anaesthetic is given (normally via a thin tube called a cannula that is inserted into the back of the hand), a team of people are monitoring her constantly.

This team is crucial: they are working closely together and are sometimes standing for long periods of time, performing meticulous work within the confines of a woman's pelvis, which is a tightly packed place containing lots of different organs and structures.

When you're under general anaesthetic, you're given drugs to help with any post-operative pain or nausea. When you wake up in the recovery room, you will be assessed to see how you're feeling and any medication adjusted accordingly. Once you're comfortable, you'll be transferred to a ward – perhaps within a day surgery or short-stay unit – to recover. Usually, this can be quite quick but, again, everyone is different.

Lots of observations are taken in the immediate hours after surgery to check your recovery, and you're encouraged to try and drink and eat a little afterwards. The nurses will want to know whether you have been able to pee afterwards, as you can't go home until they know your bladder is working properly. Sometimes it can take a while for the bladder to start working again, which occasionally requires the insertion of a urinary catheter for a day or two – sometimes longer if work has been done on the bladder itself. Very occasionally, a woman may go home with a catheter – you can read more about this later in this chapter.

The gynaecologist's perspective

Endometriosis surgery can be diagnostic, potentially 'see and treat', or planned 'elective' surgery where you know the likelihood is that the endometriosis is more complicated. The uncertainty about what you'll find is the biggest challenge with surgery.

Whilst all women referred for a laparoscopy will see a gynaecologist in the outpatient setting prior to their surgery, it's important to realise that the surgeon who does the laparoscopy may not be the same gynaecologist who they saw in the clinic. This is all to do with the NHS centralised booking systems for surgeries. In some circumstances the surgeon will have not had the opportunity to see any of the patients on their list before the day of their operation, so they may feel concerned about whether the patients will have been prepared appropriately; from a physical, medical point of view, emotionally, and from an educational point of view, with a full understanding of why they're here for the surgery.

Hopefully, by this point you will have a full understanding of what the surgery involves and what is happening but if you do have any questions or queries, make a note to ask your surgeon.

If the surgeon discovers that their patient has endometriosis, if it's superficial disease, the surgery is usually straightforward. The surgeon will either be excising it, or burning it away with diathermy (see page 72). Most surgeons will 'see and treat' simple disease. If not, the patient may be asked to come back and have another surgical procedure, or may not be treated and instead offered medical management.

A number of surgeons find that the most unsatisfactory part of their job is how the NHS is set up for them to see their patients after surgery. What's frustrating is that the patients have just come round from their anaesthetic, maybe they've managed a drink or a sandwich, they're awake, but they're often a bit drowsy, and struggle to remember what was said. Sometimes, patients don't even remember anything about what was said to them immediately after their surgery.

Before the NHS became so busy and short-staffed, patients would be invited back for a check-up about four to six weeks after their surgery, with the opportunity for a discussion about the operation, as well as to find out how they were getting on. Unfortunately, surgeons don't have that opportunity any more so it can be useful to ask for a copy of the letter that your surgeon sends to your GP.

Most patients are offered an appointment to come back to clinic maybe six months later, to see if the surgery has helped or not. Even if the surgery has helped, it is important the patients have had the opportunity to talk about what was found during the surgery properly, and understand what was done, as well as ask any questions.

In an ideal world, most surgeons agree that they would like to see their patients pre-operatively with an endometriosis specialist nurse, who the patient would have seen before the surgery. And the same nurse would phone them after their surgery – to check that they understood what happened and how they are getting on. Sadly, many hospitals won't have a specialist nurse – and far less have a specialist nurse who has time to phone all the patients who have had surgery.

Types of Surgery

There is a lot of debate about the type of surgery that is done to remove or 'destroy' the endometriosis, so it's worthwhile taking a moment to explain the differences:

- Ablation – means to destroy or remove tissue, and in this instance it is typically achieved by burning off the disease, using either diathermy (a tool that uses an electrical current to burn) or laser to 'vaporise' endometriosis lesions.

- Excision – is cutting out areas of disease. This means that deep deposits of endometriosis can literally be cut out. This type of surgery is more likely to be used for deep disease, including complex surgery where disease has infiltrated organs like the bowel. We're looking in more detail at bowel surgery later in this chapter.

In general, which method of surgery used will vary depending on the type and location of a woman's endometriosis. Your gynaecologist may use both ablation and excision during your surgery. Excision rather than ablation is usually recommended to treat endometriomas to preserve as much of the ovary as possible.

Unfortunately, even if all endometriosis tissue is removed, relapse of symptoms may occur and up to 30 per cent of women have further surgery within five years. This may not be what we want to hear – we want surgery to be a cure after all – however, we need to be realistic and consider it a treatment rather than a one-off cure.

Women's experiences of surgery

Let's hear from women about their surgeries – what were their experiences and what tips do they have for others going through the same thing?

Whilst diagnostic only surgery can be necessary – particularly if the surgical team are not in a position to deal with complex disease, find something unexpected, or it is emergency surgery – it was frustrating, explains Saskia, to have to wait for a second surgery. 'I had that laparoscopy, and because it was not a planned surgery, they didn't do a great deal, so I got put back on the waiting list for another lap to be treated properly.'

We've seen what a puzzle endometriosis can be, and whilst it might feel frustrating to wake up from one surgery to be told you will need another, it is right for a surgeon not to operate if they have any concerns. They may need to have the right people in the operating theatre to do the operation, for example, a colorectal surgeon may also be needed, so severe or deep disease may not be able to be treated at the same time.

Some women spoke of how much better they felt after surgery, even within quite a short time period. Scarlett tells us 'I remember waking up and after the first two or three days thinking "I feel so great", how bad had I been feeling before? – I think I knew I'd felt bad, but it was only when you feel well that you realise how bad you'd been feeling.'

Sometimes women end up having surgery again within a short period of time, which may be to treat new disease or deal with scarring (also known as adhesions). Emily found this was very successful. 'He booked me in for another lap, which was six or seven months after the first one where he did excision and after that, I felt fantastic, within a week I felt better and had more energy than I had done. He said there wasn't much there and interestingly, where it had been lasered off, it hadn't come back.'

For the woman herself, surgery is about much more than just the procedure itself – there's also the recovery, the risk of complications, time off school, college or work and missing out on social life, exercise and normal day-to-day life. This can be very frustrating. It can also take its toll emotionally, as Scarlett found when she had made the decision to have a hysterectomy, but was also offered another laparoscopy instead: 'If I've just had four other surgeries, why wouldn't I have to have another surgery? He wasn't really offering me anything different from anyone else and of course when I told him that I'd been bleeding and the pain when I went to the toilet, he said to me, we need to do an MRI and at this point, I just burst into tears and said I can't, I don't want anything other than my (hysterectomy) surgery.'

Most surgeries for endometriosis – even complex disease – are done laparoscopically. Very occasionally, women end up having open surgery – called a laparotomy. This means there is a larger cut in the abdomen, which allows a surgeon to have more access. However, the magnification tools used in the laparoscope are not used in this circumstance, so the field of vision is different. Thea had to have open surgery to deal with a large endometrioma and disease on her appendix. 'They couldn't remove the cyst because it was too big to take out through keyhole surgery and the endo was wrapped around my appendix so they said you're going to have to come back and we'll do open surgery.'

Recovery from laparoscopic surgery

Women will be given advice by their hospital in terms of what to expect after surgery and how long to expect recovery to take – but this is guidance. After surgery, any concerns should be discussed either with the hospital or with a GP. Some of the risks of surgery include damage to adjacent organs in the pelvis, bleeding or infection.

Recovery can be varied – not only from one person to another, but from one procedure to another. No two people or procedures may be the same. But let's look at some of the advice from women as to how to manage recovery from a laparoscopy. What does Zoe recommend? 'Really, it is just about resting, not rushing, and building up your ability to walk and sort of re-inducting yourself back into society, into life.'

Don't be deceived by the small cuts. Nicole tells us, 'I think one of the GPs put it really practically for me. If you had a great big gaping wound across you, you'd realise that you couldn't do stuff and you'd realise that your stomach had been incapacitated. Well, that's it, just imagine that big scar across your stomach and you can't move because that's what you need to do, you need to rest, you need to give your body time to heal, your abdominal wall time to knit back together – because when you look at keyhole, it's just two little marks and you think, how can I be in so much pain?'

And in terms of preparing for hospital, Thea suggests to 'always pack more clothes than what you think you need. You might be in there longer. I would definitely say to ask questions. Make sure you understand what they are looking for, what they're going to do and then just as much as afterwards what are they going to do, what they found, what the step is after that.'

Olivia felt that she was treated with dignity and respect after surgery, because she received excellent explanations of what was done by her consultant. 'After the surgery, he told me exactly what he'd found, where he found it, how he'd managed it and what he'd done ... he treated me like a normal person and discussed and respected the fact that it was my body, which was just a breath of fresh air.'

Deep endometriosis and complex surgery

We've seen before that there are different types of endo-metriosis – the superficial/peritoneal type that can be widespread but doesn't penetrate deeply into organs, ovarian endometriosis that manifests in 'chocolate cysts' or endometriomas, and the deep type of endometriosis, often referred to as 'severe'. When it comes to surgery, this is probably where these definitions matter the most.

Why is this? Well, firstly the type of surgery done for deep endometriosis – disease that may have grown into organs like the bowel and bladder – is very specialised. This type of surgery, usually performed laparoscopically, was able to develop because of advances in the type of laparoscopic instruments available, one of which allowed surgeons to stop any bleeding and another which allowed surgeons to perform surgery by keyhole without losing the gas inserted to inflate the abdomen and allow for a clear view.

This multidisciplinary approach needs the involvement of a much wider team of people, some of whom are other specialist surgeons, such as colorectal consultants or urologists, and others who will be involved in non-surgical interventions, such as clinical nurse specialists or pain consultants.

If you've been referred on to tertiary care, to an endometriosis centre with a multidisciplinary team, what can you expect? Earlier, we looked at laparoscopic surgery, both as a tool to diagnose and to treat endometriosis. This second type of surgery is the 'planned complex' surgery. These are patients who've maybe had previous surgery for endometriosis so the surgeon knows the surgery is going to be difficult, or who during their planning have been noted to have possible scar tissue or disease attached to the bowel or bladder, or deep disease, or disease in places which is going to be difficult to remove without damaging other structures.

Most surgeons will discuss all complex surgical patients at a 'multidisciplinary meeting' with other specialists in advance so that they are planned and organised appropriately. The majority of patients will have been seen and given plenty of time to discuss the implications of their surgery, both with the gynaecology team and, if there is bowel involvement, with the colorectal team. In these situations, generally patients are very aware of what the surgery is likely to entail, the risks of the surgery, and have had some discussion about whether or not the surgery will or will not be effective.

Even though the surgeon knows in advance that these surgeries are going to be difficult, they will probably feel a bit more comfortable with the surgery, because they're less likely to find something that they weren't expecting. Surgeons are always hoping that perhaps the surgery is going to be less complicated than they have anticipated, but these are surgeries that are likely to be more complicated, and have a higher risk of possible complications. So the surgeon, as well as the patient, has to be prepared to deal with that afterwards, both in terms of managing the patient, breaking the news to them, and explaining what's happened to the family, if there are any complications.

Bowel surgery

We don't know exactly how many women with endometriosis end up with the disease growing next to, on, or actually in the bowel – estimates vary between 5 to 30 per cent of women with endometriosis. Turn back to the diagram of a woman's anatomy at the start of this book (see page xxi). The lower part of the bowel, which is the rectum, is the most commonly affected place. Why is this? Well, this is next to a place called the pouch of Douglas, which is the name given to the gap between a woman's uterus and the rectum. When there is disease here, referred to as a 'rectovaginal nodule', it can be very painful and is a difficult place to operate on. Why is this?

Consultant gynaecologist Andrew Kent explains: 'It is challenging surgery because you are not operating on anything that is remotely normal in terms of tissue planes.' So, endometriosis in this area can distort the normal anatomy and make it hard to see what is going on.

Sometimes this type of surgery would be a 'two-stage' process, as in the woman may have had a laparoscopy that established that there was bowel involvement. The downside of this may be that treatment takes longer, but that means, says Andrew Kent, 'That you can sit down with a patient during the time that we are 'down regulating' (i.e., on GnRH drugs) and have a sensible discussion about what we have found and done at the first operation and what the next bigger operation will most likely involve. The only thing that we cannot be absolutely specific on is exactly what type of bowel surgery will be required (in terms of removing the disease by a "shave" or a "disc" or "segmental" resection) as this sometimes only becomes apparent when we start working through the nodule. As a consequence, we consent up to and including a bowel resection and we always do the second procedure with a colorectal surgeon. Sometimes there is an excellent result from the first operation and down regulation and although we think we may need to do a bowel resection, we end up doing a "shave".'

So what might this surgery involve? The truth is that this can be very varied. If the disease is on the outer surface of the bowel, it may be able to be shaved off without disrupting the bowel. However, sometimes the endometriosis penetrates through the surface of the bowel and this can mean cutting out a small area, or, in more difficult cases, actually removing a whole section of bowel. These can be long operations, as Andrew Kent explains. 'It can be long complicated surgery which requires a certain skill set from all involved, particularly if carried out laparoscopically.'

Consultant colorectal surgeon Mark Potter explains how he plans for operations on bowel endometriosis. 'You can get a very good idea of what to expect by looking at the MRI scans. The reason for doing the colonoscopy or sigmoidoscopy, is to get a much better feel of how the bowel is internally. If I do that examination, I can get a lot of information by the feel of the way the camera goes through the sigmoid colon in the bowel – it helps with the mental image that I've got from the MRI scan to counsel people as to whether it's going to be something that we think is going to be straightforward or not.'

So what happens during bowel surgery? This is a meticulous process of dissection, 'I personally find it mentally taxing,' says Mark, 'making progress maybe a millimetre at a time to begin with. When we're doing cancer surgery, there are a few very clear anatomical landmarks that we go for once we get into the "surgical plane" and then we can get down and we know where we are. We've used that same technique with the endo-metriosis surgery, except that some of those planes, you really lose them because of the inflammatory process. So you can find the normal plane to within two to three centimetres of the endometriosis. So you might have a little gap between safe zones where you've just got to make a decision and go for it.'

Whether this means a woman ends up having endometriosis shaved off the outer surface of the bowel, or ends up with a bowel resection, is very specific to her case.

What happens when surgeons come across something they haven't seen before? Andrew explains: 'With the complicated or rare conditions in medicine and surgery, you will occasionally come across something new or that you've not seen before. This is where two surgeons working together is particularly useful and where your training and experience is important.'

Many women worry about ending up with a stoma (colostomy or ileostomy) from bowel surgery, which is uncommon. A colostomy is where one end of the large intestine (colon) is brought through an artificial opening on the abdomen (stoma), through which faeces flow. An ileostomy is the term used to describe a similar opening from the small intestine, specifically the ileum. A pouch is placed over the stoma to collect what usually passes out through the rectum and anus (see illustration on page xxi). Very occasionally, women have a temporary colostomy as part of their planned surgery, because it has been recognised that it's necessary to allow the lower bowel to have a period of rest to heal. It is extremely rare to end up with a permanent colostomy after endometriosis surgery.

Thea had a planned temporary colostomy as part of her bowel surgery. 'They made it very clear that was the procedure because the part of the bowel that I had removed was basically my rectum, so I had to have the bag in order to let that part heal.' How did she find living with a colostomy?

'It was bearable because I knew it wasn't permanent. I knew it wasn't going to be forever. A lot of people said to me about how I just got on with things. I had it for eight months and then I had it reversed.'

Whether a woman has a stoma or not after bowel surgery, many women talked to us about how it can take a while for the bowel function to settle. The rectum has an important function, to store waste until you can get to a toilet – if you have all or part of the rectum removed, the body needs to adapt to no longer having this part of the bowel. This can result in some changes to bowel habits including:

- Urgency: needing to find a toilet quickly.

- Frequency: needing to go to the toilet a lot.

- Feeling like you need to go to the toilet but can't.

- Not being able to differentiate between wind and faeces.

- Occasionally, episodes of leakage or incontinence.

Whilst these symptoms, which are sometimes referred to as 'anterior resection syndrome', can sound quite alarming, they usually settle well over time. This can take up to a year. However, it requires patience and can mean a woman needs to adapt her life around them. Women we spoke to who had undergone bowel surgery for endometriosis talked about how they had to work out which foods exacerbated their symptoms, and which foods helped.

The other aspect of bowel surgery is that it can feel quite isolating. It's important that women seek advice and support, whether this is from clinicians or from other women who have undergone similar procedures.

Hints and tips for recovering from bowel surgery

- Drink plenty of fluids.
- Avoid caffeine and alcohol.
- Plan your meals carefully, avoiding foods that you find aggravate your bowel. This may take some time to work out what that is for you.
- Carry some supplies, such as wet wipes, any medication you might need (such as antispasmodics, pain relief, medication for diarrhoea or constipation) and a change of underwear.
- Consider obtaining a RADAR key for disabled toilets – you can order these online at Disability Rights UK (see details in Resources, page 219).
- Talk to your employer about any issues you are having in getting to work or coping at work.
- Discuss any concerns with your clinical nurse specialist, GP or consultant.

Women's experience of bowel surgery

Madison had a bowel resection and tells us how she managed afterwards: 'I changed my diet quite considerably to make it easier on my bowel and recommendations from friends that had gone through similar surgery.'

So what does that diet involve for her? 'I drink lots more water to keep hydrated to help the bowel move freely and eat plenty of fruit, green vegetables, good amounts of protein and fibre. I avoid starchy pizza, heavy breads. Things that were too heavy, too processed, tended to clog the bowel up and made it almost constipated which then can make you a bit swollen, but if you're taking care then you can manage what's going through the bowel, it means that you can live very normally.'

How would Madison describe bowel surgery? 'Bowel surgery is quite an intense procedure in terms of recovery and it takes quite a few months to recover from, and the learning process of understanding when you need to go to the toilet, the sense of feeling that you need to go to the toilet is very different after the bowel surgery. No one really prepares you for that.'

What has been the impact of this surgery for Madison, both in the early days afterwards and also now, some years on? 'I remember very clearly not being able to drive very far in the car for the fear of needing the toilet. For the first few months I really was restricted in terms of where I could go and what I could do, and my bowel movement is probably never normal again but it becomes normal to you, the new process of how you go – but you can get through it very well and adapt very quickly to having a new sensation in that region.'

How's Madison doing now? 'Although it was emotionally and physically challenging going through the surgery, it's the best thing that I ever did. I now live a very normal life and often even forget that I had the surgery.'

It's important to know that every woman's experience of bowel surgery is unique, and that seeking information and support from your team – that is, your clinicians, as well as your own support network – is vital.

Urological surgery

Surgery on the bladder, ureters and kidneys is rare. When endometriosis affects the urinary tract, the organ most commonly affected is the bladder itself.

What can you expect if you have endometriosis on the bladder? Similarly to the bowel, there may be endometriosis on the outside of the bladder, or it may have penetrated through the bladder wall, so surgery can either involve removing a small area of disease or occasionally removing part of the bladder (a resection). Normally when this happens, a catheter will be left in place for several days up to a couple of weeks, to drain the bladder whilst it heals. A catheter is simply a tube, held in place with a small balloon inside the bladder, which drains urine into a collection bag.

If deep disease has affected the ureters, it's important to assess whether this is affecting one or both kidneys, which is done by performing a CT IVU (CT intravenous urogram). This looks at how the whole urological system is working, and how urine drains from the kidneys through to the bladder. It enables doctors to see if endometriosis is stopping urine draining through the ureters. If there is any blockage, a small hollow tube called a kidney stent may be temporarily inserted under general anaesthetic to help keep the ureters open until surgery can be performed.

Hints and tips on urinary catheters

If you're going home with a catheter – whether this is due to bladder surgery or to urinary retention following surgery – you'll be given detailed instructions from the ward, along with any supplies that you need. Here are a few hints and tips:

- Follow the ward instructions carefully – one of the main risks with catheters is the risk of infection and it's important to follow what they tell you to do exactly.

- Ensure you know who to call if you have a problem with your catheter – this could be the ward, the urology team or a district nurse.
- Ensure you drink plenty of water – between 1.5 and 2 litres a day.
- Be aware of the warning signs of infection – cloudy, foul-smelling or bloody urine, fever, lower back pain, nausea, vomiting or generally feeling unwell are all important signs that you should seek help urgently.
- Eat a healthy diet with plenty of fruit and vegetables to avoid constipation.
- Keep the catheter area clean and follow instructions regarding showering and bathing.
- You can get catheter straps and stockings to hold up leg bags and make it as comfortable as possible. You won't be able to wear tight-fitting clothing whilst you have a catheter but it's important to get dressed and resume gentle activities as you recover from your surgery.
- You can go out with a catheter as normal but take care and always follow the advice of your doctor.

Possible complications of surgery

It can be hard to acknowledge that occasionally, there are complications from surgery. When surgery is more complex and difficult, there is a greater risk of complications – including damage to other organs, such as the bladder or bowel.

However, it is important to note that complications are very uncommon. That said, complications are the surgeon's biggest concern and it would be wrong to avoid talking about these because although they are rare; they can be life-changing to that person.

It's important that women experiencing any complication are treated quickly, kept fully informed and supported. It's also important to note it can be traumatic and emotionally draining, aside from the physical aspects.

Beyond surgery

> *I always say listen to your body. The patient knows their body. The women are their own experts in the disease and how it affects them.* – Wendy-Rae Mitchell, clinical nurse specialist

Women spoke extensively about 'joined-up care' and this, ideally, is what multidisciplinary teams are about. As Amy describes, this is about so much more than surgery: 'In terms of going to gynaecologists and specialist centres, I haven't experienced very joined-up support. Information on how to manage it as a chronic condition has always been very lacking. It's been dealing with the here and now and focusing on this surgery, but not living as best as you can with this disease.'

Is surgery the way to get better?

As a woman with endometriosis about to undergo surgery, you might be asking, do I really need to have this surgery? Is it definitely going to make my pain better? These are difficult questions to answer with a disease that is very specific to each patient, and where little is known about how it progresses. As a result, there is limited reliable information about the effectiveness of surgery for endometriosis.

On the one hand, it is almost impossible to conduct well-designed clinical trials to evaluate the results of surgery. On the other hand, the results of surgery are influenced by endometriosis type and extent, by the experience of the surgeon, and so on.

Nevertheless, based on the evidence from a few key clinical trials, laparoscopic surgery for endometriosis, to remove or 'destroy' the disease, is still recommended by national and international guidelines to improve painful symptoms.

Whenever a woman with endometriosis is considering embarking on surgery, we recommend that she should discuss the possible benefits, risks and complications of surgery, the possible need for further surgery (for example, for recurrent endometriosis, or if complications arise), and the possible need for further planned surgery for deep endometriosis involving the bladder, bowel or ureter.

Furthermore, as we discussed earlier, relapse of symptoms may occur after surgery and up to 30 per cent of women end up having further surgery within five years. Some women combine surgery with hormonal treatment (with, for example, the pill) following the operation – it is thought that this may prolong the benefits of surgery and manage symptoms.

Consultant gynaecologist Dominic Byrne explains: 'If you have a very young patient with relatively severe disease, it may be wiser to tolerate the disease to some extent rather than run the risk of surgery at a very young age. Some of my patients are just teenagers and that will influence the decision. Also the concept of, if you take away minor disease, it prevents it becoming serious disease is not fully accepted because the pathophysiology of endometriosis is not fully understood. Some people think that peritoneal disease and severe disease may actually have a different mechanism of development. In the past, it has been assumed that less severe disease will progress to more severe disease. That may not be true. It may be that severe disease develops more acutely and it has a different pathway and minor disease might fizzle out or change. There is a lack of understanding of the basic science of the pathology, meaning we cannot predict what is going to happen if you do or don't intervene. That knowledge is missing.'

Hysterectomy with endometriosis

In Chapter 1 we looked at the myth about hysterectomy being a cure for endometriosis. So why do some women still end up having hysterectomies? Well, perhaps a woman has very heavy periods as well, or fibroids or adenomyosis, or she may have exhausted all other treatment options and have chosen hysterectomy, alongside removal of all visible endometriosis, as the most appropriate option for her.

'Hysterectomy' is a term used to refer to removal of the uterus, but there's more than one type of hysterectomy:

- Total hysterectomy means removal of the uterus and cervix.

- Total hysterectomy with bilateral salpingo-oopherectomy is removal of uterus and cervix plus removal of the ovaries (oophorectomy) and Fallopian tubes (salpinges). 'Bilateral' means 'both sides'.

• Subtotal hysterectomy means removal of the uterus, with the cervix left behind.

• Radical hysterectomy refers to the type of hysterectomy that may be performed for gynaecological cancers. It means that, along with the uterus, cervix, ovaries and Fallopian tubes, lymph glands will also be removed. This type of hysterectomy would not normally be performed for endometriosis.

Women with endometriosis would normally have a total hysterectomy, with or without removal of the ovaries, usually laparoscopically, although ultimately the surgery undertaken is highly personalised. All endometriosis lesions should be removed at the same time.

Making your decision

We talked to some women who had either decided to have a hysterectomy or who had chosen not to.

Chloe did not have much choice as she had very severe disease and faced a hysterectomy with a bowel resection: 'Even up to the week before my hysterectomy, I went to my GP and said, I don't know if I have fought enough, I don't know if I have tried enough to have a baby. I will be forever grateful to him for saying to me, you've got as much chance of winning the lottery as you have of having your own baby.'

Zoe was not ready to have a hysterectomy, so she chose not to. 'After I'd seen the clinical nurse specialist and had an internal scan, an MRI and a blood test, the consultant recommended that I have a hysterectomy. This is a very subjective, personal, enormous decision for a woman to make, and for me, at that time, was not something I was ready for.'

Life since hysterectomy

Vicki explains how it is hard for colleagues to understand how she is now: 'I'm a surgeon and I work with surgeons, and we expect people to be better after surgery, that's the basis of what we do and if you're going to believe in your job, you have to believe that – and it isn't necessarily the case. I am better but I'm not right, and I certainly don't have the energy or the capacity that I used to. I'd say for the first two and a half, three years, I was still having quite a lot of pain of various types and I still take eight Paracetamol a day. I don't need a TENS machine or heat pads any more, so that's better. But I do have days where I know that I've eaten the wrong thing, and it's not quite right and I still have problems with sexual intercourse intimacy, so I'm not back to normal. Or even what you might think was normal for 45. You know, biologically I think it's quite a bit of my body that's more in its fifties or sixties and I don't think my colleagues understand that.'

It is a huge decision to make, and Chloe was disappointed that there was no pre-operative counselling for her: 'I had a pre-op appointment, but one thing that really got me pre- and post-op was that, I know cancer is hideous and I could never imagine how it must feel to lose your breasts, but if a woman has to face losing her breast through a mastectomy, they have counselling, or they are given some support, but there is none of that for a woman who loses her womb.'

Scarlett is making sure that she lives life to the full now. 'The one thing I promised myself after my hysterectomy was that if I was going to go through with it, I made a deal with myself that I was going to have an amazing life, so I'm just going to take advantage of every opportunity and do everything I can to help myself and everything I can to help other people – that was my promise.'

Menopause in women with endometriosis: Questions and Answers

Women with endometriosis often have lots of questions about the menopause. They will sometimes experience menopause symptoms much earlier than women without endometriosis as a result of surgery, or treatment with GnRH agonists ('temporary menopause'). Let's take a look at some of those questions:

Q: What happens to a woman's body during the menopause?

A: When you enter the menopause, whether that is naturally, due to drugs or surgically, your hormone levels will change. Natural menopause happens over many years, so hormone levels change slowly and your periods may take a while to stop, whereas with surgery or drugs, your hormone levels change dramatically quite quickly. Most women will experience menopausal symptoms. Some of these can be quite severe and have a significant impact on your everyday activities. Common symptoms include: hot flushes, night sweats, vaginal dryness and discomfort during sex, difficulty sleeping, low mood or anxiety, reduced sex drive (libido), and problems with memory and concentration. If you are below normal menopause age, you'll normally take HRT to replace some of the oestrogen lost, reduce some of these symptoms and protect your bones against osteoporosis.

Q: What happens to endometriosis when you enter the menopause?

A: Endometriosis usually gets better as you enter the menopause. We think that this is a result of markedly reduced ovarian oestrogen production from the ovaries. Scar tissue can, however, be left and so some symptoms may remain.

Q: What does HRT do to endometriosis – will it cause it to return?

A: There is not enough evidence to say whether or not endometriosis will come back when using HRT. As HRT contains oestrogen, it could theoretically stimulate any endometriosis but many women take HRT and do not have a recurrence of endometriosis.

Q: What sort of HRT do you take after a hysterectomy?

A: The lowest possible dose to relieve symptoms should be used. An oestrogen combined with a progestogen (or tibolone) is recommended because of the theoretical risk of 'unopposed' oestrogen treatment leading to malignant changes in any residual endometriosis.

Q: How will I feel during the menopause – will this be any different because of endometriosis?

A: Menopause experiences are the same as for women who do not have endometriosis.

Q: Do women with endometriosis face an increased risk of ovarian cancer in comparison to women without endometriosis?

A: The majority of women who suffer from endometriosis never develop ovarian cancer. Although several studies report a higher ovarian cancer risk, current evidence suggests that the overall likelihood of you getting ovarian cancer at all remains low, so you should be aware, but not be worried, about the impact of endometriosis on your ovarian cancer risk. While 1.3 per cent of women will develop ovarian cancer in their lifetime in the general female population, this proportion is still under 2 per cent in women with endometriosis. Thus, although there is an increase in risk, your lifetime risk remains low and is not appreciably different from women without endometriosis. To put it in perspective, as a female in the general population, your risk of breast (12 per cent), lung (6 per cent) and bowel (4 per cent) cancers are still higher than your risk of developing ovarian cancer. Certain types of ovarian cancer are more commonly associated with a history of endometriosis. These endometriosis-associated cancers tend to be picked up at an earlier stage and carry a better prognosis. There is no clear evidence so far that transvaginal ultrasound and/or blood CA-125 measurements can pick up these cancers early, or that risk-reducing surgery to remove the ovaries can save lives. To reduce your risk of any cancer, women are advised to try to have a balanced diet with a low intake of alcohol, exercise regularly, maintain a healthy weight and not smoke.

Q: Is it possible to have endometriosis after the menopause?

A: Endometriosis after the menopause is rare and, if it is suspected, it should be managed in an endometriosis centre. Post-menopausal endometriosis is usually treated by surgery (GnRH agonists and progesterone appear to be ineffective in post-menopausal endometriosis). Aromatase inhibitors are sometimes used to improve symptoms when surgery is not possible, or as a second-line treatment for recurrences following surgery.

Q: How can I help myself to feel good during and after the menopause?

A: Your GP can offer treatments and suggest lifestyle changes if you have severe menopausal symptoms that interfere with your day-to-day life. Eating a healthy, balanced diet and exercising regularly – maintaining a healthy weight and staying fit and strong can improve some menopausal symptoms.

Chapter 3

The right care in the right place for you

I tell you there are when you well up …
there are moments where people sit in front of you
and just say 'you've changed my life, because for so
many years I have had this type of treatment and it
just never really worked and now … the pain has
completely gone. We have that story frequently,
because during surgery we literally go everywhere
and take all the endometriosis out and if they
recover well, then the women with very severe cases
feel their life is transformed and so you get these
fantastic stories. Then there are the fertility patients
who have given up on getting pregnant, and we remove
the disease and then the patient conceives, without any
assistance whatsoever, those are real achievements,
but they are sort of personal achievements, you
are the only people in the room to see that, it is
wonderful. That is the driver for continuing to
fight to do these things well, when everybody or

*the system might be dragging you down, you have
to have some motivator. That is the motivator.'*
– Dominic Byrne, consultant gynaecologist,
President of the British Society of Gynaecological
Endoscopy (BSGE)

Care pathways for women with endometriosis can be
complex on several levels. Firstly, the disease itself
sometimes cuts across different hospital departments
as endometriosis can go beyond the gynaecological
organs. Secondly, as we saw in Chapter 2, the surgery
for it can be very challenging – it is not easy to treat and
sometimes further treatment is needed. Finally, it takes
many years of training and a passionate interest in the
field to develop the services and skills required to treat
endometriosis.

This chapter sets out the level of care that women with
endometriosis should expect; how to navigate the system
to receive that care, and some of the experiences of women
and clinicians as recipients and deliverers of the 'right
care' for endometriosis.

It is true that the priorities and thoughts of women
receiving care aren't necessarily always aligned to those
of clinicians. Both groups, however, passionately want
and strive for either delivering or receiving the best care:
patient-centred, high-quality care in the right place, and
at the most appropriate time. You could be forgiven for
thinking, well, surely this is easy? But it is not. That doesn't
mean we all can't strive for this, but we need to take a long
hard look at the options and the pitfalls.

We can set out the challenges of delivering a suitable and sustainable care system to women, as well as the experiences of women receiving that care. In doing so, we will pinpoint the essential elements of care for women with endometriosis, identifying best practice as well as areas that are currently less well resourced.

Not all women will have access to some of the health professionals we interviewed, such as gynaecologists who specialise in endometriosis surgery, clinical nurse specialists, colorectal surgeons with experience of endometriosis and pain medicine specialists. And, not all women will need all of these elements in their care. However, it is important to know what can be available. Sometimes women won't have all of these health services close to them – it's not unusual for women to need to travel out of their local area to receive some of the more specialised services required to treat more complex endometriosis.

The challenges of delivering the right care to women with endometriosis

Remember back in Chapter 1, we discussed the problems women face in getting diagnosed? Well, the challenges of delivering the right care start at this point, because for some women, trying to obtain a diagnosis for their symptoms can be really difficult. It's not meant to be like this and is very much unintended, however, we cannot ignore the sometimes circuitous routes that women navigate, sometimes over many years, to be diagnosed, so let's have a look at a couple of those routes:

The 'Accident and Emergency' route

A number of women that we interviewed had ended up in their hospital A&E department when their symptoms first led them to seek medical help.

I actually passed out at a golfing range and hit my head on a boulder and that's why they took me to the hospital, because I lost my vision so, had that not have happened, I probably wouldn't have even ended up in A&E so they wouldn't have even scanned me.
– Madison

Madison went on to have emergency surgery and endometriosis was diagnosed – however, some women are unlucky enough to end up in the emergency room repeatedly, where their pain may not be taken seriously. Amanda told us: 'I ended up in A&E a couple of times and they didn't take it seriously, saying, "just take some painkillers, you've got heavy periods" and sent me home.'

Occasionally, an emergency admission can result in a different diagnosis before emergency surgery reveals otherwise. This happened to Saskia, who was initially told her pain was due to suspected appendicitis. 'I'd been having pain on and off for a little while and I ended up in A&E a few times and it sort of just went away each time. Anyway after a couple of days I had emergency surgery for what they thought was my appendix. Afterwards when I woke up, I still had my appendix but also I had a name for this thing that had been causing me all this pain for such a long time and that was, you know, a really powerful thing, so it was a rubbish way to be diagnosed but I'm glad that it happened.'

The non-gynaecology referral route

Other women we spoke to had been referred to a specialty other than gynaecology, such as gastroenterology, urology or colorectal. In some cases, this led to a number of different tests – lots of them – and a delay in the diagnosis of endometriosis.

And it is entirely understandable how a woman might get here. It would be great if endometriosis could kindly just restrict itself to the 'gynae parts' – but sadly this does not always happen. This is a disease that involves itself with other organs very easily –sometimes the bowel, and also occasionally the bladder, the kidneys, the ureters (see illustration on page xxi) and even the diaphragm. This is clearly not a disease that is sympathetic to the way hospitals are structured.

The non-gynaecology route means that a woman can quickly get to understand lots of different specialties within a hospital, and often undergo many tests – but this is generally not at all helpful if you have endometriosis. A woman may end up with a colorectal consultant who understands endometriosis, or they may just end up with the rather intimidating 'bowel prep' and a colonoscopy (camera looking up your bottom) and no diagnosis.

This is probably the single most frustrating route to enter down, as Amy describes:

'I was seeing gastroenterology for about two years and then they diagnosed me with IBS, which I knew was wrong, which was a bit weird actually because I really wanted a diagnosis and then I got one and then I just thought, that isn't it. It was really strange.'

Amy ended up in and out of hospital and saw lots of different doctors. 'I went to every hospital department going – neurology, gastroenterology, the breast clinic, the dietician, the eye clinic, infectious diseases, but never gynaecology.'

The cost of this route is immense on every level – physically, emotionally, financially and socially.

Seeing the GP

A GP, or general practitioner, has a very difficult job – to make an assessment, diagnosis and agree a treatment plan for a huge range of different problems in just 10 minutes. That might be okay for a straightforward problem, but for something like endometriosis, this is a very hard ask indeed. Basically, this is extremely unlikely to happen in one appointment.

Why is this? For a start, pelvic pain is a very common symptom that could be caused by many things and often it can be a case of ruling different things out. This can take time and repeated appointments. Secondly, there is no specific test for endometriosis. There is no 'endometriosis' blood test and scans are only really useful in the diagnosis of some deep disease. Endometriosis can only be definitively diagnosed by laparoscopic surgery, biopsy and 'histology' (the examination of the tissue with a microscope in the laboratory) of the endometriosis, which is an invasive surgical procedure that occurs somewhere further down the line – it is rarely the first step for women with endometriosis. Women may end up having their symptoms treated – sometimes with painkillers and/or hormonal contraceptives – without ever being told that it may be endometriosis, even when the GP may well have noted endometriosis as a possibility.

Some women were told by their GP quite quickly that their pain and symptoms may be endometriosis. Nicole said, 'She was lovely and said, "I don't think it's anything to worry about, we'll do the usual tests just to rule out anything, but just looking at your history, I think you've got endometriosis." And I was like, oh wow, what's that? And so she told me what it was, but she wasn't 100 per cent sure, so she'd like to refer me.'

The crucial point here is that Nicole's GP told her she may have endometriosis – not certainly, but it was a possibility – and she explained what it is. This type of early communication meant Nicole quickly had a possible cause for her symptoms. With the necessary information, you are able to discuss with your GP what the potential treatment options may be, and decide together how your symptoms will be managed during diagnosis – based on you as an individual and your personal requirements.

Unfortunately, some women can get stuck in this early stage for a long time, even years, whereas others pass through the system fairly quickly – it is the cause of an enormous amount of frustration for women and doctors alike. As Amanda told us, her GP continued to tell her that painful periods were normal. 'When I did go there, say with painful periods, heavy periods, they'd just say "oh you've got painful periods, it'll settle down" and I was never offered any investigation work.'

Some women end up seeing lots of different GPs in an attempt to find out what is wrong – and sometimes this may involve lots of different treatments, different diagnoses and a lot of frustration – but you remember when you finally see someone who listens, as Beth explains. 'I had the IBS treatment, the UTI treatment, all of that, but I finally got to a good GP who was actually the psychology doctor at the University Health Centre. She talked to me, realised I was struggling but it wasn't psychological, it was physical. She said, "I am really sorry you haven't been referred to Urogynaecology or Gynaecology yet, I'll do that for you now."'

There is a lot that can be done to help this process. A useful start could be using pain diaries or using a mobile app like *Clue* and taking these findings back to the GP after a couple of months, or writing down your symptoms and how they affect your day-to-day life and taking this to show your GP. There is an example of a pain and symptoms diary on page 47.

Vicki used this pain and symptoms diary from Endometriosis UK when she visited her GP for the second time. 'When I had seen a bit more of the pattern, I then did the symptom questionnaire available on the Endometriosis UK website. I went back and I said, "I think it might be endometriosis, although it isn't a kind of textbook description of it, it does fit with some of the bits that I've seen recounted on the website," and so she said, "Yes, it seems reasonable, what would you like to do about it?"'

'The most helpful thing I've found,' Sophie tells us, 'is to summarise my own medical history and take it to them so that you're not having to say the words yourself, so you don't waste time, and get your point across.'

The relationship between GP and patient is an absolutely crucial one – some women noted that they did not have the confidence to question their GP when they were younger but wish they had been able to.

Lucy makes a useful point when she explains the importance of having the right approach when speaking to your GP. 'You have to realise that they (the doctors) are people as well. They don't intentionally want to mess up or miss things. If you go in there all headstrong and abrupt, demanding stuff, you're probably not going to get it, whereas if you have a conversation with them and respect the fact that they've been through medical school and university and have X number of years of experience, and persuade them to go down a different track, you're more likely to get on with them. I've never really had a GP say no because I've just talked to them. And respected that they have qualifications.'

The GP perspective

We are not experts, we are generalists and I think sometimes people lose track of that. – Dr Angie Gurner

It's worth bearing this in mind – we shouldn't expect all GPs to know a great deal about endometriosis as it is just one of many illnesses that they encounter and they may not come across it regularly. Since some GPs will have little exposure to gynaecology issues, it can be very useful to ask the receptionist who the gynaecology lead is in your practice – most GP practices will have one. Even when you see the gynaecology lead, this is not necessarily straightforward because women present with a range of symptoms, as Dr Sue Chorley explains: 'Well, if it's cyclical pain, I would typically ask: have they got pain before their periods? Does it go off a little bit when their period eases off? Have they got pain on intercourse ... or bleeding after intercourse and pain? But there's lots of women that I've seen that don't fit into that typical textbook description and have pelvic pain the whole time.'

The other aspect to consider with regards to your GP is that their role has changed dramatically in recent years. In the past, GPs spent a lot more time on emergency care, whereas today they spend much more time on long-term conditions and diseases that arise from changes in the way we live our lives. Dr Angie Gurner explains what it is like being a GP today:

'In some parts, standards have improved and the whole idea of communicating with the patients and the patients sharing decision-making, all that has improved. But I think the experience of being a GP has become undoubtedly more stressful, more managed by outside external pressures; national, local and driven by patients as well. So we feel quite boxed in sometimes and that is also balanced by a lot of pressure around costs. A lot of anxiety around complaints, which in 30 years has changed massively. So it's a very, very different job. And a lot of it was very acute, we saw completely different medicine, we saw a lot of people out–of–hours, we did our own out–of–hours, we saw people we know having heart attacks, strokes, acute asthma. We deal with very little acute medicine now. We are dealing with very tightly managed chronic disease, but we are also dealing with a lot of lifestyle-related disease and mental health issues. Not mental health in terms of acute psychosis, but people with stress-related symptoms, anxiety and depression, relationship problems, family disputes, pressures at work and that takes up a huge amount of time. And so the job has changed, the medicine has changed, the pressures have changed.'

Essentially, Dr Angie tells us that being a GP is about 'problem-solving and trying to work things out and piece together the history and examination findings. One of the skills of general practice is taking a little bit of time and seeing how things evolve.' This is certainly very important for endometriosis – it would create a lot of anxiety and many unnecessary investigations if all women with one or more symptoms of endometriosis were investigated. It's important to recognise this.

Dr Angie Gurner says, 'A lot of our diagnoses are made largely on a history that we take, rather than our physical examination. Diagnostically, clinical examinations probably contribute about 5 per cent to the information that you glean about a patient and the rest is listening very carefully to the story that the patient tells you. Now that depends on skills, and I think today's GPs are taught communication skills much more effectively, but it depends on time pressures and a level of interest.'

Beyond awareness, women really appreciated it when GPs listened to them and worked with them in 'partnership'.

It was acknowledged that this can result in a much richer dialogue between doctor and patient, as Amy explains when she talks about her own GP: 'I think the good thing about her is that she will admit she knows about endometriosis, but she doesn't know everything about it. But she's been willing to learn and just sort of go with me. She was willing to refer me to a specialist centre and she's been willing to look things up and have conversations with me. She trains junior doctors and she phoned me up once and said, "I was thinking of doing some training on women's health and thinking. Why don't we do it on endometriosis, and do you want to come in and talk?" And I was like, yes!'

But time is simply not on the GPs side. Not just the time to listen, but also the time to perform routine checks such as a vaginal examination. Consultant gynaecologist Andrew Kent explains: 'GPs as a rule do not have very long in their consultation to take a history and examine patients. It also makes sense to defer intimate examinations if referral is likely.'

Both from the start and throughout a woman's journey with endometriosis, the GP relationship is a crucial one. The feedback that we receive from women is that if it is acknowledged that their symptoms could be due to endometriosis, and if they are given the option to either do nothing at all, or to explore all treatment options, or to be referred to secondary care for more investigations, they are likely to be more satisfied with their care. Not just thinking about the diagnosis, but addressing pain management right from the beginning is also essential.

Giving GPs a better understanding and awareness of endometriosis is a priority area for charities like Endometriosis UK, as Chief Executive Emma Cox highlights: 'I'd like to see increased awareness, online training and an online toolkit for GPs to use, to help them support women and reduce diagnosis time. So if a woman goes to see their GP with pelvic pain, which could be a range of things such as pelvic inflammatory disease, fibroids or endometriosis, GPs have a toolkit they can easily download, a flow chart of possible causes and tests, and a way of recording progress through this on the patient's record – and with the range of symptoms for each condition, including endometriosis, which often aren't linked together by the patient or the doctor, such as bowel problems. Explaining to the patient the symptoms they have come in with could be one of several things, and some of those things could be identified through tests, and for the GP to put them on that pathway and they go through the various stages would not only speed up diagnosis, but also engage the patient in understanding what is being done and why, and what future steps might be. And at the same time, ask them to keep a pain and symptoms diary so if there are cyclical issues indicating endometriosis, it starts to be picked up in a matter of months, not years.'

But this awareness raising would extend beyond GPs, as Emma describes: 'I'd like to see more awareness generally, as well as awareness around GPs and practice nurses. I think there's an important role for us as a patient body in helping women to recognise and describe their symptoms.'

Hints and tips from a GP about getting the best out of your consultation

Dr Angie Gurner tells us how patients can help themselves by preparing for the GP appointment:

- Know what you want to say before you go along to your GP.

- Don't tell your doctor what you think it is, tell them your symptoms and let them use their skills.

- Note important details such as the date of your last period, how long you've noticed symptoms for and what those symptoms are. You might consider using the Endometriosis UK pain and symptoms diary for this, or the one on page 47 or a mobile tracking app like *Clue*.

- Don't go in with multiple problems that are likely to be unrelated as this will limit the time your GP can spend on your symptoms.

- Be ready to tell your story.

- Don't be shy about personal details because this can limit the information and the picture that your GP gets, which might delay a diagnosis.

- Be open-minded about the next steps and avoid pre-conceived ideas. Diagnosing endometriosis may include ruling out other conditions, and depending on your symptoms the GP may want to arrange tests to ensure they are not caused by another condition.

- Do your research but be mindful of the limitations of the internet (see pp. 42–46).

Meeting the gynaecologist

It was almost like a release, you know having someone believe you, having someone say actually, we know you are struggling, come in, let's talk about how we can help you. – Olivia

If you're about to see a gynaecologist, most likely having been referred by your GP, what is going to happen? As ever with endometriosis, there is not a clear pathway even at this stage. Your GP may have suspected endometriosis, or maybe they recognised gynaecological symptoms but were not sure what it was. The gynaecologist will ask lots of questions (take your history), and will discuss possible investigations, treatments and management based on your individual case. We know that diagnosis is only through surgery, and it may be that the gynaecologist recommends a laparoscopy for a diagnosis. Or you may decide with the gynaecologist to try a medical treatment prior to surgery for a whole range of reasons, individual to you.

You might think that getting this referral, this final step, will then get you a diagnosis. Well, this may well be the case, but then again, it may not. It all depends.

Let's take a closer look at this. First, let's hear from Lucy: 'I saw a gynaecologist and he told me again that I had a water infection. And I said, "Why do you think

I have this?" And he said, "Oh, there was blood in your urine." I told him I was bleeding, there was obviously going to be blood in my wee, and he told me that I just had to have antibiotics and go home, so I refused to listen to him.'

And let's hear from Sophie how it went with her first gynaecologist: 'The gynaecologist I saw told me in no uncertain terms he didn't believe I had endometriosis. Which really upset me because I had spent a long time with the renal doctor explaining to me why I had this.'

So, if endometriosis is essentially a gynaecological disease, why is it that not all gynaecologists have the same understanding of it, and why do some gynaecologists miss it altogether? To understand this, we first need to look at the referrals process – that is, the way that you are sent on from primary care – your GP – to a hospital.

How do you get treated in the right place?

Referrals are usually made by your GP to a department, rather than to a specific gynaecologist. This means a woman could end up seeing a gynaecologist who has relatively little experience in treating endometriosis because their expertise is in other conditions.

Secondly, these referrals would usually be to a local hospital, which may or may not have a developed endometriosis service. So how do the patients that need access to an endometriosis centre actually get access to one?

At this stage, it's helpful to understand the differences between what is sometimes called 'secondary care' and 'tertiary care'. Many local hospitals will provide standard services, mainly covering superficial or less complex disease – these form part of 'secondary care'. Where services provide more specialised care, such as that provided by the multidisciplinary teams, this is usually within 'tertiary care' services. Most patients would normally be seen within 'secondary care' but would be referred on to 'tertiary care' if their disease was deep or severe.

If this sounds complicated, it's because it is – identifying the women who need to be seen by a multidisciplinary team doesn't always happen quickly, but it is really important, not only from a surgical perspective but also in terms of their overall treatment pathway. Let's now look at what an endometriosis centre is, and some of the clinicians who form part of the multidisciplinary approach.

Endometriosis centres and the multidisciplinary approach

There are lots of gynaecology departments in hospitals across the UK and some have developed specialist knowledge and experience in endometriosis, along with a multidisciplinary team. In the UK, for example, the British Society for Gynaecological Endoscopy (BSGE) currently accredits endometriosis centres, and you can see where centres are on their website (see resources section on page 219).

As its name suggests, a multidisciplinary team means that the centre has built up a team of people with different skills, and this ensures they can support even the most complicated surgery. For endometriosis, the multidisciplinary team will comprise gynaecology surgeons who specialise in endometriosis, colorectal (bowel) surgeons, urology surgeons, pain-management experts and endometriosis clinical nurse specialists.

But in terms of getting referred, GPs may not know about endometriosis centres which can mean accessing the right care quickly can be hard.

If you are looking at symptoms such as pain or infertility, there may be a balancing act – does your GP try and find the quickest referral route, or the most appropriate service? What are the woman's priorities?

GPs will often look for quick referral routes, but they are under huge amounts of pressure and face frustration; they are acutely aware that they have limited resources available to them and need to refer appropriately. Consultant gynaecologist, Dominic Byrne describes the issue: 'At the moment the challenge would be to make it a level opportunity for all patients. Patients who live in Cornwall will find me, but if they live somewhere else, they may find that they haven't got someone who would undertake this type of surgery. Also their local GP or practice nurse, or whoever they talk to, isn't aware of what can be done, so there can be a lack of referral, not because of any intransigence, just actually a lack of understanding of what's available.'

It's extremely important for a woman to ask questions and take time to consider the options at every step of their treatment, particularly when considering surgery. Although accessing the right care doesn't always happen quickly and navigating the system can be difficult in some areas, knowing what can be available is empowering. Dominic Byrne tells us he uses the analogy of cancer services to describe what should happen in terms of being referred to the right place: 'Most gynaecologists now have a fairly well-developed pattern of referral for cancer. If they looked inside someone's abdomen, saw it was cancer, they wouldn't have a go and try and remove the bits they could and then send them to the cancer team; they would just stop at that point, say this is cancer, and then send them to the specialist team. We need to try and get gynaecologists to mirror that philosophy in deep endometriosis and then more patients will be signposted to the correct place first time or at least earlier on.'

Thankfully, more of this is happening now than previously. Andrew Kent explains: 'The concept of centres for the treatment of endometriosis is slowly gaining traction but although surgery and outcomes are difficult to measure, it is possible, and some good research has been done in this area. It is important that if a surgeon is unable to treat the endometriosis at initial surgery that the patient is referred to someone who can, if this is the preferred method of treatment.'

Whether women realise it or not, the power ultimately lies with patients to demand the right services, to be aware of what 'good' looks like. But this, in itself, is also a lot to ask.

If you empower the patients with the knowledge, then actually they will drive the change. – Dominic Byrne

Hints and tips on meeting your gynaecologist

- Don't be late as you may end up with a very short appointment, or have to come back at a later date. Parking in hospitals can be difficult (to put it politely!), and sometimes it's hard to find the right ward or department, so leave plenty of time.

- Take a partner, friend or relative with you for the consultation, as their presence can be very useful. It can be hard to remember everything you've been told, and two heads are better than one for remembering. If you have prepared questions you want to ask beforehand, your partner/friend/relative can prompt you to ensure you've not forgotten anything.

- Each appointment is likely to be scheduled for only 15–20 mins (and this may include time for a physical examination) so you need to 'prepare' for your visit. You should be ready to inform your doctor about all the symptoms you have noted and be able to list them in order, starting from the time when you first noted that something was amiss. Note the names of any drugs that you have taken, or are taking, and if they have helped or not. Write notes in advance, along with any questions you might have. You might have waited several months for this appointment so it's really annoying when you remember on the way home a burning question you forgot to ask. You may well have already told your history to your GP, maybe over several appointments, and the referral letter should contain a summary. The gynaecologist will want to hear you explain this in your own words to ensure they fully understand you, your symptoms and your priorities.

- Tell your gynaecologist if you cannot understand their explanations or when you don't agree. If you do not understand what you are being told, ask your gynaecologist to repeat everything in simpler language. If you do not agree with your gynaecologist, tell them this (in a polite way!), because if you do not agree with what is being suggested, you are unlikely to follow your gynaecologist's advice and treatment, and you will be wasting each other's time. Remember that you are both on the same side – yours!

The clinical nurse specialist

One of the most important developments in recent years has been the establishment of a small network of clinical nurse specialists who provide treatment and support to women within endometriosis centres. They have a pivotal role in the multidisciplinary team as they will often be the ones who are the interface between various hospital departments, the surgeons and the patient.

'I was looked after very well,' Amanda tells us, 'because I had Wendy looking after me and she was absolutely amazing. If she wasn't there then it would have been difficult. She was just there if you'd got any questions.'

Wendy-Rae Mitchell was Amanda's clinical nurse specialist, who was there for her after she had complex surgery for deep endometriosis: 'I think it's our job to make sure that women have an understanding, a knowledge and a supporting system so they can make the right choices for them at the right time. And as with everything, things change, they will change, their situations change so again, we need to be with them on that, supporting them and understanding that what they may have thought about a year ago, might be different now. We need to work with women to enable them again to move forward with those stages.'

Nurse specialists like Wendy give women the opportunity to prepare for treatment; they also support women through and after treatment, and give them the opportunity to ask questions, to raise concerns and to look at the broader impact of endometriosis on their lives. 'The nurse acts as a link,' Wendy tells us, and that link can be to a wider network of services, such as pain management, urology or colorectal services, pelvic physiotherapy, or to counselling. It's important to know that not all hospitals will have access to all these services.

'I find it amazing to hear how women cope.' Wendy explains. 'I never cease to wonder how people get through a day or get through a period of having to wait for their surgery and then afterwards the fact that it's so lovely to see the results. You know, whether they've gone on to have children or they've gone on to live a life without pain and feel that they've got their freedom back and their independence and they've got a life; they've got a future ahead of them.'

Not all women have access to a nurse with expertise in endometriosis, but women rated it as very important to them. 'I would like to see centres all around the country, centres that are talking to each other and sharing knowledge, skills, expertise,' says Wendy. 'I'd like to see a nurse in every centre and I'd like to see the nurses work into a structured pathway where the counselling side of the work is seen as important as the procedure part of the role.'

Wendy touches on an important point, that joined-up care is about more than surgery – endometriosis can take its toll on so many aspects of a woman's life, so access to talking therapies, to services that look at women holistically, can be vital to help women achieve a better quality of life.

Zoe went to a specialist centre. 'The one positive thing that came out of that was the clinical nurse specialist who did provide the emotional support and really understood that side of things, which no one ever has – we need more of that support.'

Zoe goes on to say, 'The clinical nurse specialist spent an hour with me and took my whole history and symptoms, treatment, surgeries to date and also wanted to know about the emotional impact and how I manage, how I cope, what my strategies are, and made other suggestions that were helpful and was also available at the end of a phone line if necessary, and proactively made contact to check-in how I was. That is what women need, that is absolutely what we need, so that model absolutely needs to be replicated everywhere going forward.'

Pain management

We've already seen that endometriosis can be enigmatic, that symptoms don't always correlate to the severity of disease, and, conversely, that women with severe endo-metriosis can actually respond better to treatments like surgery.

So what can be done when surgery or hormonal treatments don't provide enough relief from enduring symptoms such as pain? Well, actually quite a lot; here we look at pain-management, clinical psychologists and physiotherapists.

Pain clinics and pelvic pain-management programmes

First of all, there are pain clinics looking at a wide array of pain conditions. Often these have been established to deal with common musculoskeletal problems such as persistent back pain but through these, it's possible to access:

- Doctors who have an interest in medicines used for pain relief – often these are anaesthetists who have a special interest in pain management.

- Healthcare professionals who deal with the psychological impact of living with pain.

- Dedicated pain-management courses looking at all aspects of living with persistent pain.

We heard from women who had found these services very helpful, but in some parts of the country there are clinicians that have taken this beyond general pain management, to provide a specialist pelvic pain service. It's important to know that these are not widely available, but in our quest to explain 'right care' to you, these are services that for some women have been extremely helpful.

The clinical psychologist

Clinical lead for pain services and consultant in anaesthesia and pain medicine, Dr Natasha Curran tells us more about her work: 'Most of the work is behavioural management to help people improve their quality of life despite having endometriosis, and particularly in our case we focus on pain. We know that pain is the limiting factor for most women with endometriosis, which limits their social functioning, their family functioning, their work function, their sex function, bowel, bladder, it can have an impact on all of those things and I guess we make sure in assessment that we ask about each of those individual things, so we get a very good sense about how her pain impacts on those things, and we don't shy away from any of those things at all.'

Natasha works with surgeons operating on women with endometriosis, so her knowledge of the disease started in the operating theatre. Natasha works closely with clinical nurse specialist in abdomino-pelvic pain, Julia Cambitzi. Together they run a pelvic pain management programme called Link, named because it's a 'link' to other things, as Natasha explains: 'The nurse is really key as a link through the whole of the service. I do things on the pain-management programme as a consultant, I also give a talk on the pain-management programme, which I think links that whole thing, that it's a medical intervention. This is an evidence-based treatment which is shown to improve quality of life and reduce the impact that pain has on people's lives. I talk about pain mechanisms at the start of the programme and do a question and answer session at the end.'

On a pelvic pain-management programme like this, women learn techniques to improve their quality of life despite having pain. This is about much more than drugs to control pain. 'It's about putting people back in control, rather than the pain controlling them, so they can make choices,' explains Natasha. 'People can get into an 'under–and–over' activity cycle so on good days, they do loads and the next day actually the pain is worse, and so they then do less, and actually over time we know that it goes, that what they can do is less. So we try and reverse that and that means that even on bad days doing a certain amount, but then on good days, not overdoing it and gradually, like a marathon, you slowly, slowly build it up so that over a course of weeks, months, years, people are able to do more. Pacing activities is key to that, so what we are talking about is you can pace anything – if sitting is a problem, standing is a problem, sex is a problem, you know, you can pace all types of activities such that they don't flare the pain. And having flare-up plans, which is very important. And then actually what to do when there is a flare-up of pain so that people then don't get into an understandable panic, not knowing what to do or what am I going to do if this happens to me. We know that if you're anxious about things or if you are worried, it can often exacerbate how one experiences it.'

So this is not about telling women that their pain is going to go away – rather, this is about finding ways of living with the pain, ways of managing it day to day and coping with it. It works alongside any medical or surgical treatment that a woman may be having. It's worth noting that this is not about quick fixes – it's a lot about coming to terms with persistent pain, and acceptance. 'We expect that everyone is going to cry in a consultation,' Natasha tells us, with great honesty. What is important is that women with persistent pelvic pain come out of the course able to do more than they did previously – whether that is getting out of the house if they've been housebound, being able to walk to the gate, or open the curtains, to running marathons or getting back to work – each step forward matters to that person.

When it comes to pacing, 'I think people kind of get it,' Shona Brown, clinical psychologist, tells us, 'but then when they are trying to do that, their mind will go "Well, I should be able to do this" or "I need to do this" or just how unfair it feels to have to plan activity more and thinking about that, so that's another thing that we talk about in the group, what is it like to try and do things in a different way. And it is some of those emotions and the sense of unfairness.'

Shona runs another pelvic pain-management programme, similar to Link, that women attend for six mornings, covering areas such as the impact of endometriosis on sex. Women find it really helpful to meet other women in the same or a similar position, she tells us. 'I think there is a focus on adjustment, and we use the word acceptance a lot in the group and in the individual sessions I do'.

'It was only the other day someone said to me "acceptance, that's a big word", and it is. And I think there are sometimes misconceptions that come with that. You might think I am just resigning myself to living with endometriosis, or it means liking living with endometriosis; that's not really what we are meaning. The Latin derivation of the word acceptance is "take what's given", a willingness to take what is given and to try and have the best kind of life you can with that. I think often women feel quite stuck. It's such a horrible diagnosis and they are not really sure how they can move forward with the things that are important to them. I think there's a "coping strategies" bit of the group, but there is also a "getting your head around it" bit of the group and sessions.'

Few women currently access this type of course, but they can be extremely helpful in coming to terms with living with pain and symptoms from endometriosis.

The physiotherapist

A number of women have found pelvic physiotherapy helpful in terms of managing symptoms such as painful sex and pelvic pain by working on the pelvic floor. 'It has changed my body and my mind,' says Lucy. 'Of course I'd have painful sex when my pelvic floor was rock solid from years of pain and tension.'

What does pelvic physio involve? Basically, this is about working on the pelvic floor muscles, which may have been indirectly impacted by both the endometriosis itself and any surgery to treat the disease. Pelvic physio involves working on any 'trigger points', which are sensitive or tender areas within a muscle that can cause pain. Whilst this is not widely available on the NHS, some women have found it very helpful in managing their symptoms. You can find more about organisations that can help you find a women's health physiotherapist in Resources (page 219).

Chapter 4

Personal relationships, sex and friendships

It has a massive effect on the people around you and must be very wearing for your partner because life is not normal for them either, because you can't do things, you can't make plans, you can't just go out to restaurants when you want to, because you're in pain. – Madison

Depending on how endometriosis affects you, it can have a significant 'ripple effect' on those around you – not just to partners or immediate family members but also to friends and colleagues. That can be challenging – you may not be comfortable talking about it with others, or indeed they may too feel discomfort as you talk to them about what is a very personal and hidden disease.

But women's networks – particularly your intimate relationships, family and close friends – can be an essential part of how you manage your disease and after all, it will impact on their lives too; they're in this together with you. How does that impact relationships and what can be done, both to help partners and loved ones understand, and to enable them to help you too?

Partners

'It's very different from being in a relationship and finding out you've got endo, to having endo and trying to find a relationship. I suppose it's like that with any illness, really,' Scarlett tells us. New partners and what to tell them can be a source of great anxiety for women with endometriosis. So, you're wondering what to tell someone you are dating, and at what point do you tell them?

Well, it very much depends on you – if endometriosis is having a big impact on your life at that point in time, it might be hard not to tell them. But sharing this information with them can also give them the opportunity to support you, as Sophie found: 'I was just in a new relationship at the time I got diagnosed, which was really difficult, having conversations about whether I may or may not be fertile at that time. Luckily, I had a supportive partner and I continue to have that supportive partner, who has been a massive support. I don't think I would have survived it all without him. He is my rock. He goes out of his way to make sure I am okay.'

Partners can be really caring and supportive towards women, so taking the step to talk to new partners about it is important, but not easy. 'I think it is hard,' Nicole tells us. 'At what point do you say when you're dating, this is what I've got, this is what it means? I don't know the prognosis, the long-term prognosis, because it's an unpredictable disease, I don't know what it will mean for us. 'But he stood by me and he's been lovely,' Nicole says of the boyfriend who later became her husband.

However, every relationship is different. Just as it can be hard for a woman to adjust her lifestyle around illness, or to change expectations as a result of symptoms, so it can be hard for partners to adapt, and, unfortunately, endometriosis can place a strain on relationships, as Poppy found out. 'He told me that he was leaving me because of my ill-health, because he could no longer cope with worrying about me every single day, and that he was no longer taking care of himself. He had seen me going from being such an independent, outgoing person to having no motivation, no interest in anything.'

Sometimes women find that they need time being single, as Lucy explains: 'I was just so battered by this that I couldn't do it, so I split up with my then boyfriend, because it wasn't fair on him. I had to be single to realise what I was feeling and to try to soften myself, rediscover what I did and didn't like doing, to adjust to this new person that I'd become.'

Fortunately, many partners are able to adjust around the changes endometriosis can make to the lives of women and themselves. This can take time and mean that they too need support and understanding from others around them, such as family and friends.

Some women reported that their partners made special efforts to support them when they weren't well, as Saskia's partner does: 'I've got my partner who I've been with for 13 years now; we've been together a really long time. She's been with me all through the diagnosis and when my endo was at its worst and she's just amazing. She'll bring me things in bed when I can't get up and she'll make sure we've got food in the house and the housework is done if I can't pull my weight. She is there to help out and just is somebody who understands.'

As well as being supportive and understanding during and after any treatment, another way partners can help is to go along to appointments. Lucy found that her current long-term boyfriend was particularly empathetic because he also has health problems. 'I'm lucky that my boyfriend has a medical condition as well, so he understands when you go to the consultant.' He knows what to do to help her during flare-ups or after surgery: 'After surgery, he'll happily look after me. For example, he brought me straw-berries and cream and sat me in front of Wimbledon, so that was nice. It's just simple things like that that actually make a lot of difference.'

Some partners help out with lifestyle adjustments, such as supporting their partners through making changes to diet or exercise regimes that they may find helpful, as Daisy's husband does: 'He's very lovely about saying, well, if you need to, join the gym, or do this, just go and do it. He's always been there for me because we've been together forever, so he knows exactly how I feel without me having to say anything, so that's good.'

Whilst women sometimes identified that their relation-ships had suffered – or perhaps even ended – partly as a consequence of their endometriosis, others noted that they had grown closer.

I think endo has meant our relationship is stronger. My husband is amazing … he does so much for me and expects nothing in return. We're just a very good fit … we work despite the endo because he has made time to go to the Endometriosis UK information days, to come to appointments, to understand, he's seen what physically happens to me, how many hours I spend in the bathroom. He absolutely 100 per cent believes me ...

We talk about the future a lot, there are a lot more conversations that have to happen when you are chronically ill, a lot more planning, a lot more closeness to make it work well. I also don't see why it shouldn't bring you closer, you go through something bad, emotional and testing together and come out the other side, there's something bond–strengthening in that. – Beth

Sometimes seeking professional guidance and support for both of you may be helpful. Wendy-Rae Mitchell talks about her role as a clinical nurse specialist, supporting women with endometriosis and their partners. Here she tells us about her work with one couple prior to surgery:

I spent about 45 minutes talking to her and then we talked about where we're going to go from here with the pathway. I said, 'Would you feel this is the right time to bring your partner in?' And she said, 'Yes, that's fine.'

I brought him in and he sat down and I said to him, 'Thank you for coming in, we've had an opportunity to have a good talk about how your partner's feeling about her surgery, but I am just wondering how you are, how do you feel about this?' And he looked at me in utter amazement and he said, 'No one has ever asked me that before.' And I said, 'Well, I'm asking you now, because this is your time.'

I could hear the emotion in his voice and he was able to talk about his frustrations about not being able to do anything practical to help when she is in pain, the fertility problems … the guilt and shame he has about them not being able to have a child. It's not all about her, but how he feels. So there's lots of emotions, it's not just the one person … it affects the whole of the family.'

When healthcare professionals have the opportunity to involve partners in discussions about treatment, it can be enormously beneficial for both the woman and the partner.

What happens to relationships when endometriosis impacts upon a woman's ability to work? We'll be looking at work in more detail in Chapter 7, Adjusting life. Some women described how supportive their partner had been from a financial standpoint. Amy tells us: 'After my second surgery, I had about five months off work. It was like I was having a breakdown, ten years of being really sick just caught up with me. I needed to take time out and he just took all that financial pressure on himself and never once complained or showed it, and he's always super supportive and lovely.'

> ## Hints and tips on what to say to partners about endometriosis
>
> - Don't feel under pressure to talk about endometriosis until you feel ready to – do what feels comfortable and natural for you in terms of talking to your partner.

- Do plan what you might say; don't feel you have to go into lots of detail but be prepared to answer any questions your partner may have, or give them further information about useful websites, leaflets and information.
- Think about ways that they can help and support you, for example, coming to an appointment, attending a support group with you or an information day.
- Involve them so that they can better understand your endometriosis.
- Be honest with them – after all, they are in this with you and will want to understand and support you as best as they can.

The impact of painful sex

It feels like you ought not to be having intercourse, although you do, so you have it in your mind that actually the pain wants you to stop, but you still want to be having the intercourse. It's a really stressful thing to go through. Luckily I've got a really supportive partner and it's never been an issue. – Sophie

One aspect of endometriosis that can affect women is that some parts of sex, such as penetrative sex or orgasms, may be painful. This isn't a symptom that affects every woman but it can be very distressing, both for women and for partners. Some women unfortunately describe severe pain with sexual intercourse and some women stop having sex for a period of time. Before surgery for deep bowel disease, Madison says, 'It was really unbearable, it just completely put me off even wanting to go there because I couldn't bear it, there was nothing enjoyable about making love at all, it was just unpleasant and I was scared to do it because I didn't want to hurt.' After her bowel resection, Madison was able to have sex without pain.

Other women explored trying different positions to see if they were less painful. Sophie says, 'I've found certain positions to be more comfortable, at certain times I've had to completely say no, but we have a good routine checking that we are both okay during and after sex.'

Communication with your partner at all times is essential. 'Perhaps the hardest thing for a partner to realise is that it's not about them,' says Lucy. 'When sex is painful then no, you don't want to have sex. It's nothing personal, and there's no magic pill that'll take it away. It's simply the way that we feel. The feeling of rejection is really hard for a partner to take, and I have no advice what to do. Apart from keep talking, and find other things that you enjoy doing together.'

Some women found it hard to discuss painful sex with their doctors, as it can be an embarrassing topic to raise. However, doctors are used to discussing intimate and personal issues every day in their work, so it can be helpful to know it's normal for them to deal with sexual problems.

Being single with endometriosis

Not all the women we spoke to were in relationships, but some had noted how the physical symptoms of endometriosis had meant that they weren't ready to deal with a relationship. Scarlett tells us: 'It wasn't that I didn't ever want a relationship, because it's something I wanted more than anything, but I think because I was always so down from the pain and the depression, it took all of my energy. I didn't ever really want to prioritise it, I just didn't have the energy for it.'

Being ready for a relationship, having the energy to date and meet new people can be challenging, but the symptoms – and notably the difficulties associated with painful sex – can also affect a woman's confidence.

I think it's had a massive impact on my confidence in terms of meeting someone, and although I've been in serious relationships, long-term relationships, there's no doubt in my mind that endo has undermined my confidence in myself as a woman, as an attractive sexual woman deserving of a healthy, normal relationship, a loving relationship. – Zoe

We all deserve to have people who love us and support us. Sometimes it may be helpful to seek professional support from doctors, or for women to look at other ways to find support or practice self-compassion, like those described in Chapters 6 and 7. Some women found that a period of time being single gave them the time and space to work out what they needed next, as Poppy describes. 'It's nice to share things with someone but it's also nice to do it myself and to know that I have the capabilities to do it.'

Whatever stage a woman is at in terms of relationships, it's important to know who is there to support you. So let's take a look now at other people who may be in your own support network.

Family and friends

I'm really very lucky to have the friends that I have. I know exactly who would run towards me when others would be running away, that's one positive that's come out of having endo. – Lucy, talking about her friends

Whoever it is that women can turn to – and that might be anyone, from a close family member, to old friends, new friends, neighbours or colleagues – there is someone there who will understand, perhaps not all you are going through, but at least some part of it. Having an understanding person with you during good and bad times both deepens and strengthens many relationships.

Who is in your personal support network? It's important to know who you can turn to – perhaps your close friend is great at listening when you're feeling low, or your parents help by bringing you a meal when you aren't well enough to cook, or your brother is good at phoning you when he knows you're going through a tough patch? Whoever it is and whatever they do, these people are your incredible support network, and they are invaluable. Let's hear from women about who their supporters are and what they do to help them.

I have a friend. I've known him for quite a long time but recently, over the last year or so we've been chatting because he suffers with anxiety and depression and he

really helps me, he can tell from my text messages if I'm
having a really bad time, so he'll try and distract me.
– Olivia

Olivia's friend not only identifies with her challenges, because he faces his own health problems, but also he knows her well enough to know when she needs support, which is excellent. Lucy talks about her mum: 'We went for a birthday meal once when I was really bad and I was just lying in the back of the car with a hot water bottle and she was saying, just see how you go, we can always go home. Mum is really patient.'

When you're having a bad day, just having someone to acknowledge that and be kind and thoughtful goes a long way. Being able to be honest with loved ones also gives them the opportunity to understand exactly how it is for you. It's not always easy to be honest with people, but it can be hard for others to gauge how you are really feeling. Zoe explains: 'I think, the more open I've been able to be, the more they've understood. They know that this is part of me, who I am and how I am, and that it's very up and down and that there might be times when I can't make such an occasion or I'm not up to it. And they understand and that helps.'

This takes away some of the isolation felt with symptoms that are not immediately visible to the eye and means that others are not only able to offer help, but also can understand when arrangements have to change at a moment's notice, which can be frustrating for all involved.

One of the aspects women found hard with some friends or family was that there isn't always a 'quick fix' – long-term health issues can be very hard for others to understand, if they have neither had them themselves, nor already been close to someone else with them. Saskia has found that some people do lose patience: 'I think some people lose patience with you, they're all sympathy for a certain amount of time and then it gets to the point where they're like "Oh, are you not better yet? It's been going on for a long time." Or, if it's on your mind a lot, because it's a constant day-to-day thing so you talk about it a lot – and if you are constantly talking about how rubbish you feel then people don't necessarily really want to hear that. People get tired of what you're going through.'

Not everyone will 'get it' – and it's important to acknowledge that. It doesn't necessarily mean that they're not supportive, it may just mean that they don't understand it. It was really encouraging to hear that many family members and friends made great efforts to understand, if perhaps they didn't really know what it meant to start with. But then, often women themselves didn't understand it to start with, including Scarlett: 'I felt like I could never really have an honest conversation with my family about my situation, because I didn't really understand it myself. When I understood it, they understood it – then you can open up to people around you. I feel that really can take the burden off you.'

Some women found they were more isolated in certain situations. For example, Beth found that, at university, a lot of students were simply unaware of chronic health problems like endometriosis. 'They'd seen, perhaps, their grandparents being ill but a 78-year-old person being ill is very different to a chronic illness in your twenties. It's not expected at this age – you're meant to be invincible. I think I was really shocked at how unsympathetic some people were. I think I learnt, though, that the friends that I do have now are good friends, that I will have for life.'

Overall, it can often be the small things that people do that help. Women mentioned so many things that their supporters do – family, friends, neighbours and colleagues – if you're supporting a woman with endometriosis, or you are a woman with endometriosis who is struggling to ask for help, here are some of the things women found helpful:

I think I've been very lucky that my mum's been so supportive and calm and understanding and has equipped herself with information, done the research and has been there throughout this. – Zoe

I went (to my appointment) with my mum, my dad and my husband, and as I went in to see the consultant I said, 'I'm really sorry, is it okay if I bring in my mum, my dad and husband?' And I can always remember him saying: 'Bring in as many people as you want, because the more people you have to support you through this, the better.' – Olivia

My brother, he's a man of very few words but when I was ill, he was an absolute rock, he would just come and tell me silly things. He doesn't want to know any of the details at all but he is usually the one who says to me 'Oh don't be ridiculous, you can't do that as well as that, you're doing too much.' He's just very calm and he's really good. – Daisy

I went to see my dad and I got quite upset. My dad said, look, we will take it together, we'll work at it just like we've always worked at it, that's the important part. My mum used to come round and clean my flat for me, my sister used to come and clean my flat for me ... they used to come and clean, I'd be lying in bed and my sister would be cleaning my bathroom, they'd be saying 'Right, Poppy, do you want to come up for dinner? If you don't want to come up for dinner, I'll bring dinner down to you so you don't have to stand and cook.' Or my mum would be saying, 'Do you want to come to the shopping centre, we'll go and have a drink.' Just to get me out of the house. I think it's those little things that they do, as well as being there for support. It's just a level of understanding that they have as well and they've never doubted me. I think that's huge. – Poppy

Managing work relationships

Some people at work just don't get it, they think 'Oh she's working from home again, why what's wrong with her?' You get that anywhere, don't you really? No matter what condition you've got. – Nicole

If trying to explain the impact of endometriosis to friends and family is hard, trying to get colleagues to understand may be even harder. What can you do about this? Well, firstly it's important to work out how much you want to, or can, tell colleagues. This depends almost entirely on your relationship with them. We have heard from women who have very understanding bosses, like Nicole: 'My boss is really good and he's a bloke so, he was a bit like "Oh dear, what's this?" And then he came back the following day and said, "My wife's friend's got it" so I think it helps that you have an understanding boss, because some days I can come in and say "actually, I've had enough today, can I go home?" '

Establishing a rapport with your boss where you can discuss endometriosis and explain symptoms that people cannot see is not always easy. Equally, it can be hard for other colleagues to understand. For many women, they're likely to have a mixture of colleagues, some of whom 'get it' and some who remain unaware. Sophie has found this in her work: 'Some colleagues have been really supportive, some haven't really wanted to know about it, others want to know more.' So gauging who you can talk to at work and what you're comfortable saying to them is essential.

Madison worked in a team with people who would come and look after her when she wasn't well and needed help. 'They were quite supportive and they knew that if I said that I wasn't feeling well and I was going to the toilet – because quite often the pain would come on so severely that I would tell them, 'I don't feel very well, can you just come and check in the toilet?' because I pass out. I worked with a close team and actually everyone knew what was happening and people were quite supportive.'

Colleagues can be a tremendous source of support when you're not well, so spending time explaining endometriosis to interested people at work can be very useful. We'll look in more detail at how to manage work itself in Chapter 7, Adjusting Life.

Chapter 5
Fertility

Endometriosis can be associated with difficulties becoming pregnant, but even women with severe endometriosis can still have a baby naturally. Indeed, it is estimated that 60–70 per cent of women with endometriosis are fertile and can get pregnant spontaneously and have children. Of the women with fertility problems, a proportion will get pregnant after medical assistance – either surgery with removal of the endometriosis lesions or assisted reproduction technologies (e.g., IVF). It is important to remember that having endometriosis does not automatically mean that you will never have children – rather, it means that you may have more problems in getting pregnant. And, if you're planning on having a family, it's a good idea to try 'sooner rather than later' (now considered to be before or around the age of 30) but this always depends on life circumstances.

Why endometriosis may impact fertility

Women with endometriosis can take longer to become pregnant and can be less likely to conceive than women without endometriosis. It also appears that the more 'severe' the woman's endometriosis, the more likely it is that she will have difficulty becoming pregnant. Thus, women with deep endometriosis tend to have more difficulty conceiving than women with superficial endometriosis. We don't really understand why this happens. It may be because disease has distorted a woman's anatomy, meaning that endometriosis has directly affected her reproductive organs. Endometriosis can develop both on and within the ovaries, which could impact the way eggs are released from the ovaries, or it could affect their implantation in the uterus because the uterine lining is different in women with endometriosis. In addition, because we don't yet fully understand why women have endometriosis, it could be that the inflammatory nature of the disease directly impacts fertilisation or implantation of the embryo. Scarring, or adhesions, can also affect a woman's fertility.

Infertility

Many women will be concerned about their fertility when they first hear that they have endometriosis, but not all women's fertility will be seriously affected by it. Some women find that they can become pregnant easily and maintain a pregnancy to full term, whereas for others, it is much more of a problem. Why is this? Well, although we don't know for certain, we know that there are some risk factors with endometriosis that may mean a woman's fertility is more likely to be affected. Let's take a look at some of these:

- Endometriomas, or 'chocolate cysts' on the ovaries, can be a feature of more severe disease, and may damage a woman's ovaries. This could impact egg quality and result in lower levels of egg reserves.

- Deep 'infiltrating' endometriosis or severe disease can sometimes mean all the pelvic organs are stuck together (called a 'frozen pelvis') with lots of adhesions.

- Disease in or around the Fallopian tubes, including adhesions, is of particular concern because it can damage or block the tubes. This can also result in embryos becoming implanted in the Fallopian tube, causing an ectopic pregnancy. This is an emergency situation that may cause severe pain and always requires urgent attention.

- Multiple surgeries to treat endometriosis can impact a woman's fertility. This can be a difficult balancing act, because surgery to treat endometriosis can improve fertility, however, the invasive nature of surgery may, over time and after repeated surgeries, impact on a woman's ovarian reserve. This may be because surgery to remove endometriomas often involves removing part of the normal ovary to try and prevent them growing back again. Surgery can also cause scar tissue called adhesions. It's really important that you discuss any concerns on this with your consultant prior to any surgery so you can weigh up which course of action best suits your priorities at that point in time.

It can be reassuring to know that the majority of women with endometriosis have superficial disease and although this can be associated with infertility, many women with superficial disease will be able to get pregnant naturally.

Excision or ablation of superficial endometriosis (not involving the bowel, bladder or ureter) can improve the chances of a woman becoming pregnant naturally if they are having difficulty trying to conceive. But, there is still not enough understood about the relationship of endometriosis with infertility, and why surgery can be helpful.

Endometriosis surgery to improve fertility

Surgery for endometriosis-related infertility aims to remove any endometriosis and adhesions present. In women with superficial endometriosis, laparoscopic surgery leads to better pregnancy rates, but in women with deep endometriosis, no well-designed studies have, as yet, looked at the effect of surgery on pregnancy rates. There is also considerable debate about how large ovarian endometriomas in women with endometriosis-related infertility should be treated. Removing an endometrioma may make it easier for the gynaecologist to collect potential eggs for IVF, but removing an endometrioma may also result in the removal of some of the adjacent ovarian tissue, including some eggs. So, the decision to remove or not remove an endometrioma must be carefully considered.

Do medications used to treat endometriosis improve fertility?

Medications for endometriosis (e.g., combined pill and GnRH agonists) do not improve fertility. They also take up valuable time because you can't get pregnant while you are taking them.

So, we've established that, overall, women with endometriosis may be more likely to have fertility issues than other women, with certain risk factors potentially increasing that risk, but we also need to note that endometriosis also increases the risks of complications, such as miscarriage and ectopic pregnancy.

Miscarriage

Unfortunately, miscarriage is a common outcome in all pregnancies, whether the woman has endometriosis or not; in the general population, one in five pregnant women is likely to miscarry.

Research has shown that in women with endometriosis this risk is increased to about one in four. This is, again, a complex area that is not fully understood, but it's thought that the conditions within a woman's pelvis, and specifically within her uterus, may affect how the uterus actually works during pregnancy.

What can you do if this is you? Well, a single miscarriage may not be considered that unusual, but multiple miscarriages would normally be investigated by gynaecology, where they may perform blood tests and scans to look for possible causes. This is sometimes when a woman is first diagnosed with endometriosis. Chloe had repeated miscarriages before she was diagnosed with endometriosis. 'Throughout our infertility journey, there were a number of times when I saw gynaecologists and asked what it could be, there was a reference to "oh, it could be endometriosis", but I was never diagnosed, it needed to be by laparoscopy. I pleaded for a laparoscopy on numerous occasions through my local hospital and I did have one booked in, but amazingly I was pregnant at that time and I had a miscarriage only a few weeks before my laparoscopy, so the consultant said, "Well, you got pregnant, so therefore we don't need to do a laparoscopy and we don't need to look at what's happening."'

If you already know or suspect that you have endometriosis, what can you do if you are pregnant or are trying to conceive? It's important to know that research suggests that women diagnosed with endometriosis who are pregnant should be monitored more closely throughout their pregnancy. This may mean, for example, more antenatal scans are performed, although there is no clear consensus as to what 'more closely monitored' means and how many additional check-ups you should expect. You should discuss this with your GP, midwife or consultant.

Unfortunately, miscarriage is not something that can be prevented or avoided. However, if you're planning on conceiving, it's important to ensure that you are in the best health possible. We know that giving up smoking, not drinking alcohol and keeping to a healthy weight can ensure that you are in the best position possible to support a healthy pregnancy.

Miscarriage is often not talked about, and the experience can be very isolating for a woman and her partner. Repeated miscarriages can be utterly devastating. It's important to seek support and advice from your partner, family and friends, or seek professional help from your GP and from other services detailed in our Resources section (page 219).

*I went to work, did my pregnancy test and it came
out positive and one of my bosses was near the toilets
and she heard me scream. I am quite an emotional
person, but not overly like that. I just couldn't even
string a sentence together and when I was able to,
I told her I was pregnant and she went, "Oh that's
brilliant news" and I was saying, "No it's not, I can't do
this again, I just can't lose another baby, it's just not
something I can do." And I didn't realise I felt like
that, I wanted a baby, but I didn't realise how it was
affecting me.* – Chloe, talking about the emotional
impact of recurrent miscarriages caused by severe
endometriosis

Ectopic pregnancy

Ectopic pregnancies are less common than miscarriages,
with around 1 in 80 to 100 pregnancies ending up as ectopic.
But, research has shown that in women with endometriosis,
this risk is more than doubled.

Most ectopic pregnancies occur in the Fallopian tube.
They can cause internal bleeding and severe pain in the
early stages of pregnancy. However, they can also cause
minimal or vague symptoms. Ectopic pregnancies cannot
be avoided and once a pregnancy is ectopic, unfortunately
it cannot be maintained. Treatment is often with surgery,
although sometimes medication is used to avoid additional
trauma or damage to the reproductive organs.

If you think you are experiencing an ectopic pregnancy,
it's important to seek urgent advice and support from
healthcare professionals. Organisations such as those
detailed in our Resources section can give you advice too.

IVF and other assisted reproductive technologies

What is available to those women who, for one reason or another, cannot get pregnant naturally? One way is with assisted reproductive technologies or ART.

ART are actually a group of techniques that may be used to help a woman get pregnant. These include techniques such as IUI (intra-uterine insemination), which involves inserting sperm directly into the uterus to aid conception. IUI may also involve the use of hormonal medication to assist the process by regulating ovulation. IVF (in vitro fertilisation) is a more invasive and involved process whereby 'heavy-duty' hormonal medication is used to stimulate the ovaries to produce lots of eggs. The drug regime is personalised and tailored towards your reproductive health. Some of these drugs have to be taken by injection, which women or their partners can be taught to do. Many people find the technique more straightforward than they expected. Taking strong hormonal medication and the whole IVF process can be physically and emotionally demanding, so it's worth planning how that fits into your life beforehand.

Regular scans show when the eggs are ready to be collected. The eggs are then collected from a woman's ovary, normally under sedation, and fertilisation takes place in a laboratory. Sometimes the process of fertilisation takes place using ICSI (intracytoplasmic sperm injection), which is where a sperm is injected directly into the egg. This may be done if there are issues with sperm quality.

After fertilisation has taken place, there is a short time to wait to see how many eggs will fertilise. After this, the embryos are graded for quality. Sometimes the length of time that the fertilised eggs remain in the laboratory will be extended to allow the embryos to develop to day 5, 'blastocyst' stage. The decision on when to transfer is very individual. Usually, one or two embryos, depending on a woman's age and the quality of the embryos, are then inserted into the woman's uterus.

ART improves pregnancy rates in women with endometriosis when compared with no treatment, but the pregnancy rates remain lower than that of endometriosis-free women. The success of the treatment will depend on many factors, including your age, the quality of your partner's sperm, how long you and your partner have had fertility problems and whether you have had a previous pregnancy. Many women may benefit from a combination of ART and endometriosis surgery. Some women worry that IVF may make their endometriosis worse but there is no evidence to suggest that this happens. Sometimes women are in the position of either having to choose to undergo fertility treatment, or pursue treatment for their endometriosis. This can be emotionally very difficult and it is important to seek support from both health professionals and your own support network.

Amanda became pregnant on her third round of IVF. She sought advice and was diagnosed with endometriosis by laparoscopy. She explains what happened after that: 'We went down the IVF route but I still had endometriosis – and lots of it – but I decided to put (treatment for) that on hold and try IVF. We managed to get through a cycle of producing eggs and we did three cycles to get my first daughter.'

How did Amanda find going through IVF? 'It's involved, you're injecting yourself with hormones and then constantly having to have scans and blood tests, hoping that you produce enough eggs, and then you don't, and they're not good quality. It's an emotional rollercoaster. My life revolved around being at the hospital, having the vaginal ultrasounds, having injections, having blood tests ... I was just in a whirlwind of wanting to be pregnant so much that my life was consumed by wanting to be pregnant, especially when all my friends were pregnant.'

Undergoing IVF is a huge undertaking, so it's important to be prepared and have lots of support in place. It is important to make sure that you discuss pain relief with your gynaecologist in advance of the treatment. Amanda also wished she had been able to access counselling after her first IVF ended in miscarriage. 'I think they have that in place now in the hospitals,' she says. There is also the financial aspect to consider. 'It's just very expensive, but the emotional side of it, I don't think until you've actually been there, it's really hard to kind of see how emotionally involved it really is.'

The funding of ART by the NHS is a widely debated and controversial area. In reality, access to funding varies considerably across the UK and there may be specific restrictions, in terms of age, previous children (including those of partners), weight, smoking status and reproductive health. Younger women with a normal BMI (body mass index) and normal hormone levels (including egg reserve, measured by

AMH (Anti-Müllerian hormone)) who don't smoke, are in a relationship where neither partner has children already and do not require donor materials (see below) are more likely to receive funding. In practice, many people self-fund for assisted reproductive techniques.

Donor eggs or sperm

Sometimes donor eggs or sperm may be needed as part of the assisted reproduction process. This can be for a variety of reasons. It may be that a woman has insufficient eggs, or poor egg quality, to be able to undergo IVF treatment without donor eggs, or the quality of the man's sperm may be insufficient, requiring the use of donor sperm. Donor sperm may also be used by single-sex female couples, or by single women, to achieve conception.

When donor materials are used, there are complex legal requirements and couples or single women would be required to undergo pre-IVF counselling to be approved for the process. This specifically looks at the rights of any children conceived as a result of using donor materials, and also offers advice and support in what to tell children about where they have come from.

When women with endometriosis require donor materials to conceive, this requires extremely careful communication.

The use of donor materials for ART is very rarely funded by the NHS and can be expensive. Details of organisations who can offer advice and support on this complex area are shown in our Resources section.

Anxieties about fertility

*People don't understand why I'm scared to get
pregnant ... I'm scared because of the pain.
Not being able to take medication. I'm scared as
I'm at higher risk of ectopic pregnancy. I'm scared
because of potentially having adenomyosis, whether
or not implantation will happen. I'm scared that if
I'm lucky enough to have a baby, I'll be in too much
pain or have too much fatigue to be able to look
after it.* – Sophie

Women expressed a range of anxieties about their fertility – from the ability to get pregnant, through the stress
of potential complications and their endometriosis symptoms both within and beyond pregnancy. Preena is one
of these women: 'I mean, I'm not getting any younger,
every year that goes on is limiting my chances, so that's
my main worry. Having a family, whether my daughter
will have it, whatever may happen next ... it's kind of a
general everyday worry, but then there's no answer.'

We talked a bit about ethnicity and endometriosis in
Chapter 1, and when it comes to pregnancy, this can be
where cultural pressures may come into play. There can
be huge family pressures for some women, and families
may not necessarily know that the woman has endometriosis if periods and gynaecological diseases are not
widely discussed. Nicole felt this pressure 'because my
husband comes from a Jamaican background, he's got
masses of aunts and uncles on his side who were always
questioning when are you having a child? So there is a

persistent pressure to do that and in the end I remember I snapped at a family party. I just turned around and said, "Actually, I don't know if I can have children, please leave me alone."'

It not only places pressure on the woman, but anxieties about fertility can also put a strain on relationships with partners. 'But I think if you're with the right person,' explains Amy, 'and the timing is right, it's something you can work through ... I don't doubt that he will be as supportive as he always has been ... ' Amy's husband has been reassuring and supportive towards her. 'He said, "If we can't, it'll be sad but we have great lives and we are teammates. It'll be okay."'

Some women found they changed their priorities as a result of endometriosis, so that they now focus more on their fertility than in their previous plans, as Beth explains: 'I always thought that I would be a career woman and family would be later for me. If I had finished my PhD now, I would be trying for a baby.'

Adoption

You may also wish to consider adoption, providing a child with a loving home and family and helping them move on in life. For some, adoption is their first choice for starting or extending a family, whilst some arrive at adoption following experiences of infertility. If you're thinking of adopting it can be quite daunting to know where to begin, however there is plenty of advice from the government, councils and charities to help you find out more.

Coping with infertility

I think perspective helps because, much as I would have loved it, I try to tell myself now that I'm very lucky to have the lifestyle that I have, and I make my own choices. That doesn't mean it will ever take away the gap that is there from not having a child to love and to care for. – Zoe

Some of the hardest stories come from the women who had had to change their hopes because of endometriosis. So whilst many women with endometriosis will be able to have children, we must pay a special tribute to those women who talked to us about what it was like to move onwards from childlessness. These women courageously shared their thoughts and feelings about infertility. We leave the final words of this section to them, with the hope that at a future date, research will yield answers and solutions that mean endometriosis no longer takes away some women's ability to have children.

Chloe hopes that women and partners will be afforded a better experience of being told about their infertility: 'I had to tell my husband on my own. He came and got me and took me to the car in a wheelchair and I got in the car and I couldn't talk to him for ten minutes because all I did was cry. And then I had to tell him what had happened. I think that's devastating for anyone, I wouldn't want anyone to be in that situation. So it would be great if people can change how they tell people that they can't have children. To me that would be a really big thing to change.'

Olivia focuses on being a brilliant aunt to her nieces and nephew, as well as putting her time and energies into her work and her animals. 'Some women, they get to the point where it's the only thing that they want and it's the end of the world for them if they can't conceive, whereas for me, I kind of accepted that and thought, right, well, what can you do instead of being a mum? And that is making sure my sister's children come first for me, so my nieces and nephew, my animals, and also working.'

Saskia is grateful that her partner may be able to carry a child. 'The thing is me and my partner are in a really fortunate position in that that she could, as far as we know. I mean, she's amazingly healthy and strong and she could have children and that's something that we will definitely look into and we just have to focus on the fact that we do have that option. We are really lucky in that respect, whereas lots and lots, thousands of other women aren't at all.'

Zoe loves time with her godchildren and friends' children, but the loss cannot be forgotten. 'I'm 43 and I think I'm starting to go through the menopause. I feel as reconciled as I'll ever be to that, and I think possibly because I've been telling myself since that early age of diagnosis that it probably wouldn't happen, the driver for me has always been meeting someone and having a committed relationship for life. I've had to accept that children may not be part of that and embrace the fact that I've been lucky enough to have three godchildren and I have friends with children and relatives with children, so that I do have children in my life. In accepting that, it does come back to that loss … loss of that opportunity to be a mother, that intrinsically feminine creativity women are meant to have within us.'

Chloe reminds us that infertility is a very hidden loss, one that for many women is difficult and pervasive, but she tries to make sure she spends as much time as possible being there for her nephews, nieces and godchildren. 'All the miscarriages, all the fertility appointments, gynaecologists ... my husband and I nearly split up twice, we got closer than I would ever care to be again to losing "us". I think infertility is the single hardest bereavement you can go through because it is so silent. And people are less accepting of a pain that they can't see, but if your rite of passage has always been to be a mum or to be a parent then you know when it's gone, it's – I can't just keep saying painful, I paid a lot of money for therapy and my counsellor said to me one day, that for me being a mum was as intrinsic as breathing. And that was a really powerful statement that she made because I think she was right. And it has taken me maybe the last year to 18 months to get a level of peace and acceptance that I am comfortable with.'

Experiences of pregnancy and childbirth

We've heard about the difficulties women with endometriosis might face in getting pregnant, as well as potential complications during early pregnancy, but what happens to them when they are pregnant? Is pregnancy different for women with endometriosis and can it affect the actual delivery? Well this, again, like all aspects of endometriosis, is very individual, but we should note that the pregnancy and birth experiences of women without endometriosis are also extremely varied.

I was amazing in my pregnancy, I had no pain for the first time ever in years. The pregnancy itself, I carried really well with my first daughter, there was no pain, I didn't feel how I felt with the endo, all drained and tired, an emotional wreck, I just felt pregnant. Yes, it was lovely that nine months. I felt good, it was a good time of my life to be honest.
– Amanda

So what can we say specifically about women with endometriosis? One aspect of this is that the method of delivery may be affected by complex surgery. Amanda became pregnant naturally with her second child within months of having a bowel resection for deep endometriosis. This pregnancy sadly ended in miscarriage, but then she quickly became pregnant again. Her second daughter was delivered by caesarean section. She tells us: 'I thought I was never going to get pregnant and I fell pregnant again and then our second daughter was born by C-section. Miraculous! I don't know how she arrived but the symptoms subsided completely during pregnancy, I felt really good, really great. When I had my C-section done my gynaecologist said my ovary was clear, there was no endometriosis, it was lovely, it was all nice inside.'

Daisy was diagnosed with endometriosis during her first pregnancy, when an endometrioma was found on her ovary. This made her first pregnancy extremely stressful and difficult because she had to have surgery on her ovary whilst pregnant, which is rare. She found giving birth, in comparison to her actual pregnancy, more straightforward: 'Actually when she was born, I was really quite relaxed, or I thought I was – because I felt like it was not nearly as bad as what I had gone through, like giving birth to her was not as bad as the rest of it.'

She wasn't expecting to get pregnant again, but she did: 'I was told I probably wouldn't have any more children, which was not a surprise, except that I think possibly because of having had the cyst removed and then breast-feeding for a while, I actually got pregnant a second time after my daughter, so I had them fairly close together. A definite miracle baby!'

Her second pregnancy was much more straightforward: 'I just felt it's amazing being pregnant in a normal way. I don't think I really worried about endometriosis because I was just, "Oh great! I'm pregnant, I'm not having periods, I'll just deal with it all afterwards."'

If you're a woman with endometriosis who has concerns about what pregnancy or labour might mean for you, you should arrange to speak to a healthcare professional, whether that is your consultant, specialist nurse or midwife.

Being a parent with endometriosis

We've looked at the potential challenges of getting pregnant, pregnancy and birth for women with endometriosis, but what are the issues that mums with endometriosis might face once a baby arrives? Many women are anxious about how their symptoms might be after pregnancy, or how it might affect their ability to look after a child. Let's first hear from women about what happened to their endometriosis after pregnancy.

The endometriosis during my pregnancy was fine, I had a straightforward pregnancy really ... The endometriosis sort of went away for nine months but then came back with a vengeance when she was born, so it was held off for all that time and then it came back really badly after she was born.
– Amanda

During pregnancy, whilst a woman is not having periods, the endometriosis lesions that were there before pregnancy will still be there, but they often don't cause symptoms. However, once periods start again, the symptoms of endometriosis are likely to return.

Nicole's symptoms stayed away whilst she breastfed: 'I breastfed my daughter and my symptoms were okay, they were really manageable and yes, I suppose you do get relief from it, and it was only when I stopped breastfeeding that it started returning. They can't really say to women "now get pregnant" because I don't think it solves the issue. I mean, you do get a bit of relief if you breastfeed – if you don't breastfeed I think it comes back quicker.'

Ava found that her symptoms did improve after childbirth. 'Having been through childbirth, the endometriosis pain has certainly reduced, but it hasn't gone away entirely. It doesn't disappear; instead it keeps coming back. What is different is that I no longer writhe around in agony. I am much more able to deal with my pain myself than I ever used to be.'

How did mums with endometriosis cope with their symptoms returning? Nicole tells us, 'I've really enjoyed having my daughter. It can be hard work in the days when I'm poorly, there's a lot of guilt. All she wants to do is play but I'm going "No, Mummy can't move, can I just give you a cuddle?" "I don't want cuddles, I want to go and paint, go outside and go to the park… " That's quite hard at times because all I want to do is sit down and you can't, so it's been hard.'

Daisy had a difficult pregnancy due to a large endometrioma on her ovary, so she feels she has been 'maybe more relaxed as a mum because of it, because I just had so much trauma'. Daisy is now able to spend more time focusing on her own health and managing her diet, but she wasn't able to do this immediately. 'There have been times I've felt really ill and I've just had to carry on, but mostly the children have been a big distraction. It wasn't really till my son was nearly one that I found the energy to go and look after myself a bit more.'

Taking time to look after yourself, seeking support from your family and friends, and doing whatever you need to do to help you cope with your symptoms are important for mums with endometriosis. We'll look further at things that women have found help them cope with their symptoms in Chapter 7, Adjusting life. Nicole copes through: 'A lot of stubbornness and determination … I'm always doing stuff, because if I'm doing things, I'm not thinking – but it has caught me out. I've had to stop in the middle of Tesco's because it really hurts. I've had to catch my breath and go, "Oh that was not nice" and obviously if I'm with my daughter, there's a bit of a look as well because Mummy's screwed her face up and she doesn't look very nice.'

Nicole finds she has to weigh up taking painkillers to manage pain, versus being able to be there as a parent. 'They say they can give me stronger painkillers but how can I function as a mum, as a parent and a wife if I'm all zonked out?' This can be very challenging and emphasises not only how important a woman's support network is, but also how tough it can be to manage symptoms when you're a parent. 'The hardest part of having this disease is when my endo is bad and my son is also not well. Obviously, I must still nurse him. I must ignore the fact that I am hurting or feeling sick because he needs me,' says Ava.

And although it is challenging, women with endometriosis who have children are always reminded just how precious and special their children are:

My daughter is my positive out of endometriosis. I've got her, you know. I will take my daughter, if I've got endometriosis for the rest of my life I don't care, but equally I need to do something to spread knowledge. I can't just sit there and do nothing.
– Nicole

Daughters of women with endometriosis

Now I have a daughter, what are the implications? ... Have I given her that awful disease that I have, is that my fault or is that just the way it is? – Nicole

We know that, although you are more likely to have endometriosis if you have a relative with it, the genetics of endometriosis are complex and it is unlikely that a woman will pass the disease on to her daughter. But all of the women we talked to that had children spoke, not only of their deep worry of passing the genetic makeup that may cause endometriosis on to their daughters, but also of their desire to ensure their children were better equipped to understand periods and be aware of what is normal, and that applied to both sons and daughters.

Ava talks about endometriosis to her son: 'My son and I are close and we do have topical conversations and I will discuss endometriosis with him in depth so that he has a clear understanding and appreciation of a woman's struggles with this disease. I think it is important because there is always the possibility that he could befriend, date or even marry someone who has it, and I would like him to know what we go through and be that support; be that rock for someone else.'

Women with daughters are particularly anxious for them, but are conscious about not projecting this worry on to them, as Daisy explains. 'I feel quite aware that I have a daughter and that one day perhaps endo will be her inheritance. I feel I will probably – the first period she has – be watching her every move and questioning her. I mean, partly in a good way, because I will know. She already knows that women have periods and it happens every month. I obviously didn't tell her that it was painful, there's obviously no point at the moment.'

With their own knowledge and experiences, however, women with endometriosis ultimately know that both their daughters and sons will have the one thing that perhaps they did not have themselves: awareness. 'That's one generation that has been educated,' says Nicole. And with that knowledge comes the clear opportunity for earlier diagnosis.

Chapter 6

The invisible effect: the emotional impact

Endometriosis is a particularly difficult condition to live with because it is an 'invisible' chronic pain condition – it's not like having a broken leg, for example – and other people struggle to imagine what it's like to live with it. In addition, this is compounded by the fact that endometriosis is a 'woman's problem', and some men (and some women) are uneasy talking about it. Not surprisingly, the 'silence' around endometriosis can impact considerably upon a woman's mental health, which we will discuss in more detail in this chapter.

Any serious physical illness, particularly any illness that may be chronic or persistent, can have a profound mental health impact, over and above the effect on someone's physical health. This is, in itself, a widely recognised phenomenon. Of course, some women with endometriosis may not experience symptoms that are chronic or persistent, whereas for others, even despite the myriad of treatments, there may unfortunately be symptoms that persist.

But the attention paid to the mental-health impact of endometriosis has been, to date, fairly small. Why is this?

Endometriosis is a disease with traits that probably make the impact on a woman's mental health even more pronounced, for example:

- Diagnosis: some women experience a significant delay in diagnosis and commonly talk of a failure to be listened to, to be taken seriously. This may not only be damaging to a woman's self-confidence, but it can lead to feelings of not being believed, or being let down and ignored. The lack of a diagnosis can, unfortunately, be very damaging.

- Embarrassment: the effects of endometriosis can cut right to the core of what it means to be a woman – from dealing with painful sex, to excruciatingly painful periods and embarrassing symptoms such as bowel problems. These can all also be deeply taboo, isolating and just not spoken about. This can lead a woman to be effectively 'silenced' and therefore feel alone.

- Treatments: these often rely on hormones and painkillers, both of which may impact mood. In addition, treatments may last a long time, be ineffective and other types of treatment, such as surgery, may also need to be repeated. There is often not a simple treatment profile and certainly not one that works for all.

- Quality of life: endometriosis may affect every aspect of a woman's life, from her relationships to her fertility, her ability to work, have a normal social life and achieve her hopes and dreams. Whilst this is not the case for everyone, many women to whom we spoke talked of a profound sense of loss, akin to that experienced with bereavement, which sometimes had a lasting impact on their mental health.

In this chapter, we will look in detail at how endometriosis impacted the mental health of women in these scenarios. We will look at what helped them, both in terms of the services they may have accessed, and also the things that friends and family or the women themselves were able to do to help deal with the mental health impact of having endometriosis.

Beyond the physical suffering of a delayed diagnosis, we cannot easily measure the real impact of treatment delays on the actual disease process (it is still unknown as to whether this is a disease that always progresses – for example, if mild disease becomes severe disease over time), or the psychological distress that has been endured. But we can reflect on what women told us. What does it do to someone to keep their suffering hidden, or not to be believed?

Madison was diagnosed in her late 20s and she talks of: 'The emotional impact during my teenage years and into my 20s when I was coping, or trying to cope with it, and then the pain before the surgery and then the worry about what was happening. The time off work, the complete lack of control in terms of my time and being off sick from work, the pressure that that brings; that was a very emotional time for me and very hard and I felt very low.'

A lack of control seems to be a common theme – how frustrating not to be able to plan or commit to being at school, work or social events. Added to this, very hidden symptoms can be hard to talk about, and therefore isolating. Amy spoke about the impact this had had on her self-confidence as a girl. 'I think probably as a young person, it impacted on my confidence. I felt like I wasn't believed, which was not a nice feeling. I didn't really feel that there was anyone I could talk to about it who would understand and it did kind of isolate me a bit, to make me feel like I wasn't one of the normal girls.'

At times, this very loss of control can lead to depression, which is what happened to Scarlett: 'I think for me it caused depression because I felt a real sense of not being in control of my life. I always felt as if I wasn't really getting anywhere. It was like the rug was being continually pulled from under my feet every single day and I just couldn't ever take some control over my life.'

The impact of endometriosis can run deep for some women. If you're a woman who has been suffering for many years, who has perhaps tried a few treatments or had a number of surgeries, but symptoms persist – and added to that is the potential impact on relationships, family, fertility and work – that can be an awful lot to handle.

Zoe has had endometriosis for over 20 years and within that period there have been times of more increased suffering, and times of less. She reflects, 'I guess over the years you become used to the pain, and your pain threshold, and how your body tolerates pain, which helps you to manage the pain, but I think in recent years for me, well, all the way through, but particularly recently, the emotional impact can just knock you for six, really knocks you sideways.'

Treatment for endometriosis focuses on physical symptoms

Since many of the treatments for endometriosis are hormone-related – and beyond that, we have surgery, sometimes lots of it – treatment in itself can be challenging. This may be especially so for the heavy-duty hormonal treatments that put women into a temporary menopause. Surgery has a different set of challenges: there's preparing for it, anticipating it, hoping for a good outcome and sustainable relief from symptoms. Then there's the operation itself and recovering from the anaesthetic, then the process of recovery from the procedure, which varies from person to person. It can be frustrating. It can also be a very emotional time.

Hospital services for endometriosis are largely set up to deal purely with the physical side of things. It is not surprising that there may be little or no focus on the emotional impact of treatment. But it would seem short-sighted to ignore this – women spoke at length about the emotional side of this disease and its treatments. Zoe, who has had five surgeries for endometriosis as well as various hormonal treatments, explains, 'Cumulatively, I think that many surgeries definitely take their toll physically and emotionally, and again all the treatment and care, it's physical, not emotional. There's no advice about how you might feel after an anaesthetic emotionally, or the impact of having that surgical treatment or time off work; it's very physically focused rather than emotionally.'

What can be done about that? We've already talked in Chapter 1 about delivery of news – sometimes women remember very clearly how they are told about their disease, even if they can't remember what they are actually told. Olivia believes this is partly down to educating health professionals: 'I think that medical staff need to be educated more in terms of how it affects patients mentally because I think they need to take extra care with how they deliver news, and how patients are supported post-treatment or post-surgery.'

The hormonal side of this disease deserves some serious consideration when we think about the emotional impact – hormones can leave women feeling very low, not themselves and sometimes unable to cope, as Emily describes: 'I can deal with being in pain or tiredness, it's when you've got them both and then when the hormones kick in and you're low. Nine times out of ten, when you're feeling horrible and you just want to throw something at someone, you know it's the hormones and you can't sort of snap out of it, but sometimes you do feel really kind of down about things.'

It can be extremely tough to deal with severe symptoms and hormone treatments at the same time – a couple of the women who we spoke to had been, on occasions, in a bad place. It's really important to talk to someone who understands when things are very difficult. We hear reports of feelings of hopelessness, despair, even suicidal thoughts, and urgent help must be sought in these circumstances.

This happened to Lucy, who has a good relationship with her mum and looks to her for support. 'I was in a really bad place and she was really, really good then. Actually I've talked to her about that since, because I didn't really want to die, I just didn't want to be awake, if that makes sense. So I did think about crashing my car when I was driving once, but I didn't because I had the dog in the boot and I loved my dog more than I loved myself at the time. I was taking Zoladex, tramadol and I was sleep-deprived, I wanted to claw out my womb. I just didn't know what else to do. So I called the doctor as soon as I got home and then I couldn't speak to tell the doctor.'

If you are in this position, or supporting someone feeling desperate or suicidal, please see our Resources section on page 219 for details of how to get help and organisations to contact.

The impact on quality of life

What happens to women when they suffer the emotional impact of this disease? We have seen some women feel very frustrated by the impact on a woman's ability to do 'normal things', the small things in life that many of us take for granted, like an evening out with friends, cooking dinner or even completing domestic chores. This may be hard to read – and we again reflect that every woman is different – but we must give voice to the hardships that some women face. Women like Saskia, who explained, 'I know you shouldn't judge your life on other people's, but you do look at what other people are doing and compare yourself, compare yourself to that and that's really frustrating that I don't have more energy or am not well enough to go out and do things that other people are doing.'

Whether this is a short-term or longer-term challenge again will vary – but it can leave women very anxious and worried – as Saskia elaborates: 'And then when you are feeling ill, not knowing how long you're going to feel ill, what does it mean, does it mean it has spread? Is it going to make my bowel worse than it has been before? Am I going to need another operation? So all of those unanswered questions and the worry that it causes, I think that's the worst, to me that's the worst.'

There may be, for many women, unanswered questions, times when you are not sure where it will end. Endometriosis may be a long-term or chronic condition for some women and dealing with persistent illness is hard. One woman, Vicki, described the impact of endometriosis as 'long–term and low' – and this may ring true for some. Whether women are dealing with acute flare-ups, hospital treatment or the persistent effects of the disease, such as bowel symptoms or persistent low-level pain, there is a risk that any of these aspects could affect a woman's quality of life and well-being.

Women told us that they sometimes had to dig deep to keep going, as Nicole describes: 'It's hard some days. You're screaming in your head, actually, I don't want to do this or do that and I'm really scared that if I just stop and say I'm not going to do it any more, what will happen? Will I just fall on the floor and not be able to get back up?'

But finding the motivation to do so can be very personal – Poppy describes what she calls her 'lightbulb moment', the time when she realised she was desperately low and needed to find a way forward: 'I remember lying in my bed and I was watching the TV. I hadn't showered for about three or four days, I hadn't got out of bed, couldn't be bothered, didn't see the point. I thought, well I'm going to be aching anyway. You know it's going to hurt, so why would I bother? I remember there was something I can only describe it as a lightbulb moment – suddenly something that just made me go, "What are you doing? Why are you doing this?" And I remember thinking, I have hit rock bottom again.'

Sometimes the first step to moving forward is accepting that life may be different, the challenges may alter what you can do, but coming to terms with those differences is a vital step forward.

A few women noted that it wasn't necessarily the symptoms that reminded them about endometriosis. Sometimes it was their visible scars that they saw every day; sometimes it was the effects on their lives – perhaps the altered career path that they were on, the impact on their relationships or ability to have a family, or the altered diets they were following. They may not have received treatment for the disease for a while but they were reminded of it. As Preena explains, 'I think about it every day, because in the morning when I get dressed, I've got a massive scar down my belly. It's there, the reminder is there daily.'

Amy is upset because it has affected her studies, where she has already achieved so much: 'I'm annoyed on so many levels. I haven't even finished my PhD, I don't know if I will. Do I just put that down to endo? I feel it's really messed it up and it feels unfair.' For Amy, this also means that she isn't doing the job she imagined she would be doing. 'Every time I go to work, I think – I actually love what I'm doing, my job, it's given me a new lease of life, but I would never have done this job if I'd been well. So, I'm always thinking about endo, not actively, but it's always on my mind.'

Not being able to forget about it appears to be quite common – even when symptoms may have improved – because of the sometimes sustained or profound impact on a woman's life. We may be better now, but what has it cost us? Daisy finds that she thinks about endometriosis a lot. 'I do a lot of research and reading about it. I just constantly remind myself why I'm doing it. Endo is in your head every day isn't it? It doesn't matter what you're doing. Even if you're feeling okay, it's still a massive part of who you are.'

Before we look at some of the strategies that women used to help themselves with the emotional impact, let's hear from some of the health professionals involved in supporting women with this disease. A small number of women receive support from clinical nurse specialists with expertise in endometriosis – nurses like Wendy-Rae Mitchell, who explains, 'My role is working with women and their families and in order to do that I work with them holistically. I see them as individuals, because the disease is so individual and I think it's really important that I sit down with them, listen to them, and hear what they have to say. Often I have to listen to a very distressing story. And I feel that they deserve the time and the recognition, because obviously there's been a lot of suffering before they've got to seeing us in clinic and then I feel it's my job to work with them to enable them to manage as best they can their symptoms and their lives.'

Women may also access support through their GP, through counselling services or through clinical psychologists. Counselling gives people the opportunity to talk openly and in confidence about their experiences, whereas cognitive behavioural therapy, or CBT, is a particular type of talking therapy that focuses on strategies to help you manage your problems by changing how you think and behave.

Lucy is having counselling and CBT. 'I think even after diagnosis just having a chat with a counsellor, to realise what you feel, because I was on so many drugs I couldn't feel anything, I was completely emotionally numb for about two years after.'

Some women have taken antidepressants to cope with anxiety and depression related to their disease. Zoe didn't want to take antidepressants and felt that that was all that was on offer to her. 'There's probably been a couple of occasions when I have been to my GP feeling incredibly low and I've always mentioned endo and the impact that that has. The immediate response after reviewing history, thinking about what might be triggering an episode of feeling low, or depressed is, well, here's a prescription for antidepressants and that's not necessarily right for everybody.'

Olivia has struggled with the mental health aspects of having endometriosis, which resulted in her having her ovaries removed at an early age. 'I wasn't offered any counselling about the removal of my ovaries. I think the mental-health side for me is a massive gap as well, you know, looking at these patients and saying actually, they could be depressed or anxious because of the fact they have this condition. They are isolated, they can't get out, so let's see if we can give them some CBT or things like that, rather than just giving people tablets all of the time. Coping mechanisms and looking at things differently is a better way.'

In an ideal world, every woman would be supported with access to counselling, to talking therapies like CBT, and to have the support of trained professionals with in-depth knowledge of endometriosis, such as clinical nurse specialists like Wendy. But what can be done when access to these services is limited? How can women adopt self-management strategies that help, both now and for the longer term?

If the women we spoke to talked at length about the emotional side of endometriosis, they also spoke passionately about a huge range of things they had done to help themselves. Not just talking to others – although this is absolutely vital – but explaining that even when life was difficult, small things helped them. We heard stories about pets – from dogs and cats to smaller animals like guinea pigs and Gordon the hamster – journeys of self-discovery and doing active things like exercise, hobbies and making choices when they couldn't do everything they wanted to. We also heard at length how support services offered by charities – particularly peer-support groups — gave women, their partners, family members and friends the chance to talk openly to others about what they were going through. These stories were so powerful.

When times with endometriosis are tough, women showed us that they sometimes got tough too – so, we hand this space over to them to tell you their tips:

When times are tough – stories of how women coped

Talking

The thing I find most challenging is mood and fatigue. I don't know if I can peel myself off the sofa, but if I stay on the sofa, that's going to make me feel worse. I should really try and go and be sociable but sometimes you just can't manage it, so it's balancing it, and knowing when the right time to do that is and when it isn't. If you can't go, pick up the phone to someone and just have a chat. – Zoe

Pacing yourself and resting

I think just breaking things down into bite-size manageable chunks, rather than seeing the bigger picture the whole time, thinking, putting pressure on myself, I have to do this, work this week, do this socially, I have to do XYZ this week, even if only one of those things are achieved, that's okay. And giving myself permission to be like that helps. And reaching out to people I've learnt is so much better than feeling alone with it, because you can just really intensify those feelings of lowness or depression. And it's hard to do that sometimes and you have to make yourself do it but it does help ultimately I think. – Zoe

I do have the days where it floors me and I accept that and I don't feel bad about it; I don't feel bad about myself if I need to have a day where I'm in bed and I don't move and I don't have a shower and I don't wash my hair. If I feel crap then I allow myself to do that because I know that that's what I need to do. – Poppy

I think the days where I rest are, 'Oh, it's almost won today,' but I am trying to turn that around into saying 'no, it's not won today,' I just get to watch lots of box sets today. So all that television that I've been missing out, that's sat on my Sky planner, today's the day where I can just get the blanket and live on the bed, so I'm trying to sort of flip it around and not get disheartened when there are days where I can't physically, where I am too physically tired to do anything. – Nicole

Being kind to yourself is hugely important — you have to do that, you have to be kind to yourself and not

judge yourself too harshly when you're in pain. And also thinking that everything passes; you might be in terrible pain for however long but just keep thinking it will actually go away, it won't be there for ever and ever, it will go away – as hard as it is to do that, and I don't think it's possible always. – Saskia

I have learned to recognise that I have low points and they're quite often associated with a flare up. I'm in a good place and I can allow myself to have those times and then move on from that.… I feel much more in control now than I probably have done in the past and I know what I need to do and where I need to achieve. I'm very good at managing my symptoms. I know when I need to take time out. – Sophie

'We do stuff when we can … '

Walking, cycling, swimming … I was even able to horse ride once I got my endometriosis under control, but just generally anything where you're moving the body and being a bit active; it's all about releasing the endorphins to help boost your mood and lift you. If your mood is boosted you generally can deal with these things a bit easier. – Madison

I talk to myself a lot in my head. I think because when I was younger and I was in a lot of pain, I'd always tell myself that I had to get up and go and do stuff, you had to go to school and you had to go to work. I never thought I'm going to give in, I'm not going to sit down and do nothing. – Daisy

I remember my mum trying to push me forward with certain things and I was like no, I don't want to do that, I'm not ready to do that yet so when I'm ready to do something, I know it's the right time for me.... I had that moment and I started to think, well, okay, how can I change this around and how can I try and make me better? Because that's what it was about; it wasn't about trying to suit anybody else, it wasn't trying to make me better to make other people happy, it was about me. You really do learn a lot about yourself and how strong you are. – Poppy

I think it made me value the important things in life, like walking the dog, or cuddling up with a TV programme or book, not going out and getting drunk or going to a club. Because those things are not enjoyable any more, I completely lost interest. – Beth

Pets can give love, comfort and routine

I made myself a nice cup of tea and I had a long chat and cry to the dog. He was great, he listened and cuddled me, licked away my tears and gave me his paw. I got myself sorted out, but I do owe my life to that dog.– Lucy

My therapy for myself, in a way, is rescuing animals. I've got six guinea pigs, so they're not difficult to look after but they give me so much pleasure and the reason I got them is I needed something to give me some sort of routine and responsibility; I need to get up to go and feed the guinea pigs. If they need some food, I'd have to go down the road to the pet shop to get some fresh air.

Little things like that keep me motivated to keeping to a routine and keeping going. – Olivia

You feel a little bit lost because you don't have a focus. I think that's one reason why my cat's been so good, because she has been my focus, you know, especially when my ex and I split up. She is the best decision I have ever made – she gets me up in the morning, she comes when I've cried, she talks to me, she is a comfort. – Poppy

The difference peer support makes

Women can receive support from the Endometriosis UK helpline, through online support groups and internet forums such as HealthUnlocked. Many women spoke about the very positive impact from attending face to face support groups:

The thing that's probably helped me the most is attending the Endometriosis UK support groups. Knowing that there were other people going through similar things to me and who I could go to and ask questions about things they had already experienced, and could advise and help me find different solutions to my problems. I definitely think the support group has prevented me from having a mental-health problem. – Sophie

Essentially, it's a safe place to talk, share and listen. We've had ladies who have had IVF, their husband has known but they haven't told anybody else, they haven't

told people that they've had five rounds of IVF that have failed, that's quite emotional. It's being around people who understand that if you arrange to do something and you can't go, it's okay, you don't feel you have to explain yourself. That's the best bit, actually. Endo is a part of every aspect of your life, but having friends with endo means that it's our "normal", and that makes it easier to live with. – Lucy

The Endometriosis UK support group and meeting other people in the same situation was an absolute lifeline and without that I don't think I'd be in this position today. – Madison

Knowing that you can help somebody the same as they can help you, just having that there I think makes such a difference. – Amanda

I stayed really upset for about a year, really upset. So I did all my own research and I joined my local support group. It was really good. I mean I went to talk to my GP as well. Far and away the support group was the best thing really. The support group – I can't sing the praises enough of that, it's fantastic and I've definitely made friends for life there. You get useful information and incredible support, I've definitely found that there. – Amy

It's really nice to see the change in women from just the beginning of a meeting to the end . When a new person comes they're tearful, they are scared and they are very quiet. They'll start talking and making bonds with somebody, or somebody says something that they relate to, and by the end of the meeting they're feeling a lot more secure and they've got hope. – Saskia

Chapter 7

Adjusting life

'Getting out there and living is really important in moving on with your life after the surgery. I think for a lot of people, the fear is that life won't get back to normal again, and it absolutely will, but you have to take control of getting yourself well and getting yourself in the best possible situation to help yourself, whilst keeping an eye on things and always questioning if things don't feel quite right and going back to get them checked. And if you exercise regularly, look after yourself and stay positive, you can move forward and get on with your life.' – Madison

We've looked in detail at endometriosis – the challenges of diagnosis, the array of treatments and finding the right care, as well as the impact on relationships, fertility and the emotional side of it. We're now going to look at how you can move forward with your life when you've had a diagnosis and treatment for endometriosis. Let's first take a look at work and careers.

Work and careers

We started to look at work in Chapter 4, where we looked at managing work relationships. Most of the women we spoke to are working, whether this is full-time, part-time or in a voluntary capacity. Working arrangements and careers take all shapes and forms and it's important to know that, however endometriosis affects you, there can be a positive outcome when it comes to work and careers. It may involve compromises, unexpected changes and indeed it may turn out that you follow an entirely different career path to the one you were expecting, but there will be a solution nonetheless. So, how do you find a way forward with work? Let's have a look at some of the aspects of work that women spoke about.

Sickness absences

Some women end up taking time off work regularly due to symptoms, whereas others find they mainly need time off after surgery. How do you tell your employer, and how do you manage this time off? Preena says, 'It hasn't impeded my career and generally when I've told employers about the endometriosis, they've been quite understanding.'

Some employers will be understanding, but what about repeated periods of absence and describing symptoms to employers, if treatments have not yet given you the relief you expected? 'It's difficult, you feel like you're disappointing people,' Saskia explains. 'Work feels at the forefront because it affects a lot of people, it's not like you can just get on with it by yourself; a lot of people are affected by whether you're at work or not and whether you're doing a good job.' Some employers, like Saskia's, are excellent. They made efforts not only to understand endometriosis, but to work with her individual circumstances so that she felt supported at all times. She says of her employer: 'I do feel at work like we're all on the same team, and that team is trying to keep me at work for as long as we can. I'm not fighting it.'

But what can you do if your employer does not understand why you're having time off work? Olivia was in this situation: 'I would get taken into the office and told: "You're ill again, do you realise how many days you've had off sick?" and it would make you feel guilty, that you're a bit useless and, because I didn't have a diagnosis at that time either, I did feel like almost I was made to feel like a liar.'

First of all, it's important to recognise that this is not your fault. Many women to whom we spoke felt very guilty about time off sick. Endometriosis can sometimes be a difficult condition to manage and it's essential to recognise that and try and find the best way forward with your work.

It's important to find someone you can talk to at work – whether this is your boss, a HR manager or another colleague – and explain to them your symptoms and how they affect you in your working life. Of course, you may be like Olivia was and have not yet had a diagnosis, which makes it even harder, not to have a name for what's causing your symptoms.

It can be useful to talk to occupational health if your work has access to this type of resource. Poppy tells us that 'We have occupational health, and they were really good at accommodating me being on light duties.' Occupational health can be a useful resource in terms of understanding exactly how your endometriosis impacts your particular line of work – after all, jobs vary widely, and whether you are working in an office or outdoors, are on your feet every day or working shift patterns, the challenges you face could be very different to those of other women living and working with endometriosis.

You may also be able to access support from a union if you belong to one, or if not, you could seek advice from the Equalities and Human Rights commission (see Resources page 219 for more details).

'My first ones weren't great,' says Emily, talking about a previous employer, 'they were when it all kicked off initially and they thought it was just one surgery, they were lovely. As soon as it started to come back, they went all funny and had their HR person do a risk assessment and asked would I be rude to clients, which was frankly insulting.' It can be hard to explain that endometriosis is not a straightforward condition – we can't predict the pattern that a woman will go through. Some women find that their symptoms are manageable for many years, whereas for other women, their disease and symptoms come back quickly. This is extremely frustrating for women, and as people can't gauge from the outside how someone is feeling, being frank with an employer is important. 'On the whole I've been fortunate,' Zoe tells us. 'I've had managers who've been understanding, who've been flexible and supportive – I've had to do a lot of educating them about the condition and the effects because there is very little out there in the public domain about the impact this can have on a woman's ability to work, or sustain a career.'

It can be hard when you're put in a difficult work situation. Some women, like Thea, end up having disciplinary action taken against them for time off sick. She explains: 'It gave me problems because I was calling in sick for two or three days every month and this was happening right up until I had surgery. I was given disciplinaries at work for my sickness. Even though it was genuine. I was given a disciplinary after I came back after recovering from an operation, because I had been off for a month, regardless of the fact that I had got a note; they just said it was because you were over the company average absence percentage. This is the routine and if you're off sick again, we'll go up to the next disciplinary level.' Thea no longer works for this employer, but her sickness absence was not well handled by her employer. Why is this? Well, it's important that employers make an assessment as to whether someone's ill health, whatever condition or symptoms they have – even if they have not yet been diagnosed – would be viewed as a 'disability'. This isn't necessarily a simple assessment, although in most cases it will be quite obvious. Let's examine this further.

Disability

There are very few conditions that are automatically classified by the Equality Act 2010 as a 'disability'. This is because for the vast majority of diseases, how they affect a person is individual and there will be huge variation, even within one single disease. One woman's endometriosis may cause mild symptoms, whereas another woman's could have far-reaching effects. There is no one pattern.

The important aspect and the only question that really matters is this: are the symptoms of endometriosis 'disabling' for you? And that means, do they substantially have a negative effect on your ability to perform normal day-to-day tasks, and is this likely to be the case for a period of longer than 12 months? This also does not mean the effect has to be every day – fluctuating conditions, such as the way Thea was consistently affected every month, are also covered.

If you're likely to be covered by this definition, this may mean that sickness absences related to your endometriosis symptoms could be excluded from any sickness absence calculation. However, the law doesn't explicitly require an employer to disregard disability-related absences in this way.

But this might be an appropriate 'reasonable adjustment' for a woman with disabling symptoms from endometriosis. Sometimes women find other 'reasonable adjustments' help them to work. Let's look at some of these.

Flexible working

Nicole explained her endometriosis to her boss, who now has a good understanding of it. She's allowed to work from home sometimes: 'I think that's what I like about having the freedom to work from home. If I really need to go and put on the baggy trousers, they can't see my baggy trousers, whereas at work, because I work for the directors, you have to wear quite smart business dress and it can be quite restrictive when your stomach is bulging.' Working from home is a great example of flexible-working arrangements, but it isn't always possible – some jobs just cannot be done from home. However, if it's possible for the type of work you do, what process would you go through to ask for a flexible-working arrangement?

Employers normally have policies in place that cover disability. Any 'reasonable adjustments' that may be requested from an employee would normally have to go through the company process. Whilst there is no guarantee that an employee will always be granted a 'reasonable adjustment', employers are required to make every effort to try and accommodate these where they relate to disability. Even though the onus is on the employer to try, it's worth knowing that it's not always possible. It's important to be open-minded in terms of working with your employer on disability-related adjustments – sometimes you can have a 'trial period' of any adjustment to see if it is workable on both sides.

It's important to remember that what constitutes an adjustment that might work for you is one that looks at your individual circumstances, what is challenging for you and what your role is. Whether that is standing for long periods of time, or working hours during your periods, difficulties with travelling and commuting or needing access to toilet facilities, the aim is for the employer to work out whether it's possible for them to accommodate that.

Saskia's employer arranged for her to see occupational health and she has a plan in place, with adjustments made to her work: 'We came up with a plan with the occupational health people and they read up a lot about endo so they knew what it was, which was lovely. It was really helpful – just simple things like whatever classroom I'm given will always be near a toilet and I'll always have a class that's got another adult in it, so that if I need to leave, I can leave the classroom.'

Changing career paths

'I've not had any issue getting to work since my surgery and medication change so it hasn't been an issue. I haven't had any time off work in the last nine years due to endometriosis,' Madison tells us, which is excellent. Thankfully, many women find that the effect of endometriosis on their working life is short-term and, following treatment, manage to get back to work and resume their careers.

But this might not be the case for everyone – some women have found themselves leaving jobs or careers because they were unable to sustain them. This can be disappointing and frustrating for women affected in this way. 'Work for me has been a big thing, having to change my entire work,' Emily explains, 'because I'm an advocate, a barrister, so that's probably been the hardest part for me.'

Aside from the emotional and financial impacts of changing your working life, research in this area has shown that the loss of working time has a significant cost to the economy (*'Impact of endometriosis on quality of life and work productivity: a multicentre study across ten countries', Journal of Fertility and Sterility*, August 2011). It can be difficult to plan sometimes, but perhaps knowing your own personal limitations allows you to be more selective in work that you look for. 'I think it's just the job thing that frustrates me, I'm definitely going down a different path now than I ever planned. Also I don't have a plan, whereas before I very much had a plan. Now I'm going day to day,' Amy tells us.

· 'Even with the jobs that I take, I have to consider if they'll offer flexible working, such as working from home, because as qualified and determined as I am, I have to be prepared,' Lucy explains, knowing how endometriosis affects her. And she acknowledges that sometimes, this might mean she undervalues her skills in the workplace. 'My boyfriend will push for a pay rise at work. I don't value myself, but if I was pushing for a pay rise I'd be thinking, oh but I might have to have sick days or go to hospital appointments, so I take that in as part of my pay package, when actually it's nothing to do with my work, it's part of me, but it's not my profession.'

One of the hardest aspects of work is accepting that priorities and goals sometimes change, but there can be other paths and roles that are both fulfilling and rewarding. Scarlett has achieved a lot in supporting other women with endometriosis, but she tells us that she has lost out in her career. 'It's affected my working life hugely, because I don't feel as if I've ever really been able to reach my potential at work.'

It's important to know your personal limits with endometriosis, and to acknowledge that sometimes adapting or changing jobs or career paths might actually better suit your needs. Whilst we know and acknowledge that it can be really hard psychologically not to be achieving what you may have set out to achieve, it doesn't help to feel guilty, frustrated or inadequate. You are doing your best and adapting to the challenges you face, so be kind about yourself and acknowledge your own skills and talents. You are unique and the world needs what you have to give!

Hints and tips for dealing with employers

- Do try and have an open dialogue about your symptoms with someone you trust at work.

- Do explain, in as factual a way as possible, what you are experiencing and how this affects you on a day-to-day or month-to-month basis.

- Share information about the treatment you are undergoing and some of the basic facts about endometriosis, explaining that one woman can be affected very differently to another.

- Try and understand the challenges from your employer's perspective as well, as endometriosis is a complex disease and can be hard to understand. It's important to recognise that your employer will have their own pressures and that they have to plan resources to get work completed.

- Be open-minded about changing your working arrangements if they no longer work for you – flexible working can be really helpful, and often new opportunities arise. You may find a career path that suits you even better.

- Seek advice and support from unions or other organisations relevant to your line of work.

- Seek support from your wider support network – whether this is your partner, family, friends or through other women with endometriosis.

- Look at any benefits available to you that may help you, and seek support from organisations such as Citizens Advice Bureau that might help advise on the paperwork for these.

- Talk to your GP, clinical nurse specialist or other health professionals about work concerns.

- Don't be hard on yourself about your own health challenges; try and focus on getting better rather than feeling guilty,

- Don't be defensive with your employer – it won't help.

- Don't assume or expect an employer to make a 'reasonable adjustment' automatically – this isn't always possible.

Exercise

Exercise is probably the best thing that helps, I started taking up running, I joined a gym.... I walk a lot, so that's helped me massively with the pain, the fatigue and the bloating as well. – Preena

Exercise forms an important part of a healthy lifestyle and is now recognised to be of benefit for many chronic pain conditions, but exercise can also be one of those areas that slip when a woman is suffering from endometriosis symptoms. However, it can be invaluable to fit in even a small amount of gentle exercise into your daily routine, such as swimming or walking.

Exercise releases endorphins, which are the body's natural feel-good chemicals; they interact with receptors in the brain to reduce the perception of pain. 'Walking and cycling and just getting out in the fresh air boosts your mood, it does help, exercise is a natural pain reliever. You feel like you really don't want to do it, you almost have to push yourself to do it because it does help, it really helps,' Madison tells us. After she had recovered from bowel surgery for endometriosis, she was also able to resume one of her favourite hobbies, horse-riding.

It can help to introduce new activities slowly if you're not used to exercising. Daisy does yoga, which she started off slowly 'because I just kept thinking, well, how will I know if it works, if I don't do it slowly?' Yoga can be beneficial both physically and mentally, as it also involves an awareness of breathing and promotes relaxation. Some women do Pilates, which works on your core muscles and pelvic floor. If you are experiencing pain in this area, it's important that you talk to a clinician before commencing any new programmes of exercise.

Psychologically, making the effort to do even a small amount of exercise can make a lot of difference, as Nicole has found. 'Some days I've only done 10 minutes – it took me longer to drive there and back than it did to actually do anything, but I think because I'd managed to get up and get there, yes, I didn't do very much, but I got there. It can be a boost to your confidence and it also means you are getting out and doing something positive, which is helpful.'

Resuming activities that are important to you is essential when you have a disease like endometriosis – whatever it is, whether it is running, dancing, yoga football or simply walking, it's helpful to exercise but know your own limits.

Diet

Sadly, currently there is no scientific basis to guide women, or support, dietary measures for the treatment of endometriosis specifically. However, we are very aware that some women find this a really important part of their own self-management plan, and it's worth talking to your GP, clinical nurse specialist or consultant about making dietary changes, if you're thinking of doing this.

Avoiding processed foods and reducing alcohol, as well as choosing fresh, naturally available foods and a wide range of vegetables is recognised as an important part of any healthy balanced diet. Many women with endometriosis try dietary measures to improve their symptom control – sometimes this approach can be successful – and sustainable.

It was very gradual. To begin with I probably just ate the same thing all the time and it just made me more and more aware of my body, because everything I did made me feel just that little bit better. – Daisy

Sophie doesn't eat gluten now, and she talked about this with her clinicians. 'When I asked both my GP and my gynaecologist about that, they said there was no scientific evidence to support that and they didn't mind what diet I went on as long as it wasn't a diet that eliminated all food groups, so I was healthy.' Why do some women find that not eating gluten helps their symptoms? Well, gluten is a protein found in wheat, spelt, rye and barley. It gives foods like bread an elasticity and chewiness. If people have coeliac disease, which is an autoimmune condition, they cannot eat gluten at all without having severe physical reactions, but there are many people who don't test positive for coeliac disease but still report sensitivity to gluten. Gluten may be problematic for people with IBS – and some of the symptoms of IBS cross over with those of endometriosis.

Some of the women with endometriosis that we spoke to said that they had benefited from a diet that helps people with IBS, which is the 'low FODMAP diet'. This is a diet that is recognised to help IBS sufferers. FODMAP refers to 'fermentable, oligsaccharides, disaccharides, mono-saccharides and polyols'. These are carbohydrates that are found in a wide range of foods, such as onions, garlic, wheat, rye, beans, lentils, milk and certain fruits and vegetables. Consider seeking the advice of health professionals, as this diet is sometimes followed under the guidance of a dietician.

Saskia found elements of the FODMAP diet helped her, but it was difficult to maintain beyond the short term. 'I changed my diet dramatically, which I started doing with the help of a dietician. I did some of the FODMAP diet where I reduced all different types of food I was eating and I just ate three ingredients for a week and then every day after that I was allowed to introduce new ingredients. So I did carrots, oat and chicken, I think, my first three things, because I could have oats and oatmeal for breakfast and then I could have carrots and chicken. After, I introduced potato. I did this for ages. I didn't notice any particular benefits and in fact I was cranky from not being able to have a bar of chocolate or cheese, I really missed food so much ... I decided that it wasn't for me – it wasn't worth it.'

Daisy follows a gluten-free diet with no caffeine, sugar and limited amounts of other foods. It can be tough to follow but she has found the benefits worth it. 'I wrote a list to myself in case I ever got discouraged because it's quite hard-core. I wrote down how I used to feel and how I feel now and it motivates me when I've needed to be. Here's my little list: my periods are better, my pain days are down to one or two a month most of the time, and the pain is less. There are other benefits like better hair, sleep and skin, less "brain fog" and more energy. A better immune system and overall increased confidence because of all this. I'm gluten-free and wheat-free, I don't have any refined sugar or caffeine, no alcohol, no soy, basically no processed foods, pretty much no dairy, very little red meat ... It's full on but it's so good.'

We hope in future that there will be more research so we can understand exactly how diet affects women with endometriosis.

Complementary therapies

Complementary therapies are normally used alongside conventional medicine as a way of coping with symptoms. They're not used to 'treat' endometriosis, rather to manage living with it. They can include treatments such as aromatherapy and traditional Chinese medicine, known as TCM. Alternative therapies are used instead or alongside conventional medicine.

Acupuncture

'Acupuncture is based upon two thousand years or more of practice. It is not magic, however, it has been described as magical by some of the patients I have treated with the meridian balance method acupuncture,' says Dr Ooi Thye Chong, who is a certified licensed acupuncturist and lecturer in integrative medicine. She tells us, 'with this style of acupuncture, pain relief can be immediate, although not permanent. One woman, Monica, comes to mind. She is a typical example of how acupuncture has helped my patients, diagnosed with endometriosis or had chronic pelvic pain of unknown cause. She has had surgeries and tried many medications to no avail. However, the only therapy that relieved her debilitating pain was acupuncture. Because of her intense pelvic pain, she often had to be wheeled into my clinic by her boyfriend, but after treatment she walked out pushing the wheelchair! Once the acupuncture needles were inserted, Monica's pain would subside, the colour on her face returned, her breathing slowed down and she felt herself again.'

When you have acupuncture, fine needles are put into your skin at specific points. Traditional acupuncture believes that energy called 'Chi' flows in the body. It is thought that if the Chi does not flow well, you may have health problems as a result. Acupuncture can be used to re-balance the flow of Chi – to restore and maintain health. Acupuncture can help relieve pain. It is thought to work by causing your body to release its own pain-relieving and anti-inflammatory chemicals (e.g. endorphins and cortisol). There is some research data that supports the use of acupuncture for chronic pain in general, but more research is needed to see it is helpful for endometriosis pain.

Ooi Thye explains her research on this area to us: 'As part of my pilot trial on acupuncture and chronic pelvic pain in women, participants reported in the focus group discussions that acupuncture lowered their pain and enhanced sleep and energy levels, as well as giving a general sense of well-being. For example, one participant reported that while she was pain-free, she was able to spend quality time with her three-year-old daughter. The pain relief afforded by acupuncture could be likened to taking pain medications but without the unacceptable side effects.'

This is a treatment that's not usually available on the NHS but private practioners are easy to find, and some women find it really helpful to cope with pain. Madison told us she found it relaxing and it gave her some comfort psychologically, whilst Emily finds it helpful for her pain: 'I had acupuncture before the last surgery and that was a life saver and absolutely fantastic, because I didn't want to have to take anti-inflammatories and take the gastric medicine with it... so I started acupuncture and it was fantastic, it was really good and I was so convinced it helped.'

Reflexology

'I don't even know if it works,' says Lucy, 'but lying having a foot rub is quite nice, and that's more of an escape from your head. The lower your stress levels, the better it is for your endo.' Several women commented on how helpful reflexology had been for them, alongside other complementary therapies. Zoe felt a range of these therapies had helped with her well-being, 'helping with fatigue, mood and feeling low'. Amanda found reflexology so helpful that she also trained as a reflexologist, a complete change in her career. She found the relaxation from reflexology, combined with mindfulness meditation, a really important way to cope with how she felt in herself.

Natural hormone therapies

Some women try natural hormones, instead of synthetic ones. Zoe has been trying bioidentical progesterone, which is a product derived from yams. Zoe explains why she decided to do this after having GnRH drugs: 'I decided I would take a year to be free of anything and see what my body did, and I tried alternative therapies and treatments. I've reached the point now where I am on bioidentical progesterone, which I've been on for about six months, with mixed effect.'

What difference did Zoe find with this? 'The bioidentical progesterone does lift the mood a little bit and makes me feel a bit more on an even keel. I had a phase of time without it for about two months and my mood really plummeted.'

Social life

I used to really resent missing out on things because of endo, because I was feeling grotty and in pain and debilitated by it. It's a balancing act, because sometimes I think if it's pain, I know how to manage that, and sometimes it helps to go even if it's just for an hour, just to see and be with people. – Zoe

Some women spoke to us about important social occasions that they had missed out on, like birthdays and weddings, or the disappointment about letting friends or family down by cancelling plans at the last minute. This was often a juggling act. Do you tell friends that you'll go out, knowing you may need to risk cancelling last minute, or do you limit your plans at certain times of the month and feel a bit isolated? Sometimes it can be a real trade off, knowing that your plans may need to change at a moment's notice. In reality, everyone has to change plans sometimes, and most people will understand how that feels.

Thea likes to accept invitations and is optimistic about being able to attend social events. 'I don't try to let it take over things. If people invite me to something, I look at the calendar and I think, oh well, I'll just say yes and then we'll see what happens and if I can go, I'll go.' Having this flexibility in approach means she doesn't often miss out seeing her friends. Being part of a larger social network is an important part of everyone's life, so it's essential to keep those ties.

But what happens if you find you are repeatedly missing out on your social life? Olivia tells us: 'Our bodies just can't keep up, so you still want to do things, you still want to have a family, you still want to go out, you still want to work, you want to go to the birthday that everyone is going to – but you can't go because you physically can't manage it. It's that barrier, not being able to do something when you really want to do it in your head.'

It's very important to recognise that important trade-off between not doing something and feeling sad about it, versus accepting the invite and perhaps trying to do something when you feel below par. Knowing what you need to do for you is very important – and sometimes that will be accepting that it's more important for you psychologically to be having that contact with others, taking that time with your friends and family, whereas other times, it'll be more important to have rest.

Don't be afraid to be honest with people in your social network – after all, they care about you and will want to support you and understand your challenges. If they don't understand about how endometriosis affects you, that could be an ideal opportunity for you to improve their awareness.

Learning about yourself and campaigning for change

*It's made me a lot tougher, going through that at 17
made me really strong. I used to say, I'm never going to
see a doctor, I'll be fine. And then it happens all at once.
I had the operation and going through that at 17 wakes
you up. I think I'm a lot less naïve to the fact that
illnesses do happen. I think if that never had happened,
I'd still be eating rubbish, I'd still be having the same
bad diet and lifestyle I was having, so in a way, it
helped.* – Preena

Despite the challenges of endometriosis, many women
spoke about what they had learnt about themselves, from
the little things in life making you happy, to the realisation
that women had strengths they hadn't previously known
about. There were some reflections that those moments of
self-awareness were really important.

'I've changed the way that I deal with things,' Poppy tells
us, 'and I now think, okay, I have a chronic illness, I will
live with that chronic illness, but I won't let it defeat me.'
Women like Poppy showed us their resilience in dealing with
challenges that endometriosis had dealt them. They'd rather
not have had to deal with them, but there was no choice,
so they're doing what they can and actually learning along
the way. 'It has, ironically, given me some more confidence,'
says Daisy, 'because I've had to work through so much stuff
that I've come out the other side. I'm grateful to it in some
ways. It sounds absurd, doesn't it? But, ironically, I don't
know if I'd ever have got this healthy without it. I think I'm
much stronger because of the horrible time I've had.'

Beyond this resilience, some women find the disease brings out in them a real desire to see change for other women, the drive to fight for progress. As Scarlett explains: 'I'm now actually getting a chance to contribute something, to write and to help people, and be vocal to help others have a better experience than I did.'

Women are honest about their suffering, but they're also keen to empower other women. 'I hope that we can reach more women and make more women aware, support women more,' Zoe tells us as she talks about the positive aspects of volunteering for Endometriosis UK. Volunteering not only increases self-confidence and the sense of accomplishment, it also means that you're doing good for others, and that gives people a lot of happiness. It not only connects you to others, but it's good for your mind and body, and can be fun and fulfilling at the same time.

'We are forming a community,' says Amy, as she talks about lobbying for change. 'Even in the few years that I've been diagnosed, you can see how it's changing and I think a lot of pressure can come from us as a community that historically hasn't been there. I think that's something that needs changing as well, it will all have to come from us.'

Women with endometriosis have a very important role, not only to speak out about the challenges of it, but to work towards better understanding in society, more research into causes and treatments and ultimately, consistently better outcomes for women.

Chapter 8

The Future

We've looked in great detail at how endometriosis is treated currently, and this alone has seen major advances in recent years with improved surgical techniques through laparoscopic surgery and a rapid increase in awareness, thanks largely to the internet and social media. Let's now turn to the future, as there are still many areas of unanswered questions and so much scope for even better treatments.

The future for research in endometriosis is clearly a huge topic but we recently tried to tease out the key issues by surveying nearly 2,000 women with endometriosis, their supporters and healthcare professionals, and asking them what they felt was important.

Perhaps not surprisingly, the top priority for everyone was to find 'a cure', followed closely by women and clinicians wanting to find out 'what causes endometriosis'. Clearly, these questions are inextricably linked – if we are to find a cure for endometriosis we need to find out what causes the condition to start with.

But first of all, we believe that we really need to better define endometriosis. Are there truly three subtypes – peritoneal/superficial, ovarian and deep? Secondly, if there are different subtypes – are there different mechanisms to explain why they occur? And thirdly, do these subtypes need to be treated differently?

Other 'hot topics' from our national survey included raising awareness of endometriosis amongst healthcare practitioners through education programmes, and improving diagnosis.

Defining endometriosis better

Over the last few years, researchers have made commendable attempts nationally and internationally to ensure that samples (biopsies) collected from women with endometriosis are carefully and accurately defined in a uniform way. This has included taking into account the wide-ranging symptoms experienced by women with endometriosis, as well as the appearance and location of the endometriosis lesions. We believe that this will significantly expedite the research efforts in endometriosis and enable researchers to perform large-scale, cross-continent studies to address the research questions important to women with the condition and the healthcare practitioners that treat them.

Dominic Byrne, the endometriosis surgeon we heard from earlier, says, 'to advance research in endometriosis you need to take a certain group of patients, patients with indisputable disease so you are sure that the population you are studying is the same. Then you need to collect everything you can from them; blood and store it; a history of the observations and findings; and look at biopsies of the tissue; and then you look for patterns.

Do the patients carry the same genetic code, does the histology show certain characteristics or biomarkers? This is the basic science and it needs to come alongside the surgical and the clinical experience and only then will you get breakthroughs. These types of scientific observation can develop into something that can be backed up by facts and could lead to someone saying, well actually, I can tell you why that happens; it's because this gene is not expressing this protein and therefore the peritoneum is not responding in this patient like it does in a patient without endometriosis.'

Professor Philippa Saunders, a scientist in the field who has researched endometriosis for many years adds: 'I think endometriosis is a disorder that is crying out for a more precise, "intelligent" approach to therapy. To me as a scientist, there is a minimum of three diseases (superficial/ peritoneal, ovarian and deep) and the research community are not actually modelling all three of them in our studies. What we need is to develop new ideas focused on identifying the best treatments for each of these subtypes of endometriosis, so that the clinicians can place better emphasis on personalised care. Personalised care will be the only way forward.'

Lessons learnt from cancer research

Increasingly we are learning more and more about endometriosis by considering the results from studies in cancer, which are much more numerous than those on endometriosis.

Whilst endometriosis is not a cancer, it does behave like a cancer: it can spread around the pelvis and 'destroy' local tissue, and is sporadic in that it affects some women and not others. We can draw some parallels in the ways cells behave in both conditions and we hope to exploit this knowledge to 'repurpose' drugs for endometriosis patients.

Deep endometriosis lesions isolated from women undergoing surgery for endometriosis have mutations (changes in the genetic make-up) in some genes implicated in endometrial cancer. Furthermore, for an endometriosis lesion to develop, it needs to 'stick', 'invade' and 'form its own blood and nerve supply' – and these are all steps that occur in cancer.

Not only are the steps in cancer replicated in endometriosis but there is new evidence to suggest that the cells lining the wall of the pelvis ('peritoneal mesothelial cells') are 'metabolically' different and can enable the steps.

Normally cells break down sugars in their mitochondria – the energy packs within the cells. Cancer cells instead switch off their mitochondria and break down sugars in the cytoplasm – the main area of the cell. This is known as the 'Warburg effect'. The cells in the pelvis of women with endometriosis also behave in this way.

For a number of years now, cancer researchers have been trying to exploit the Warburg effect to find new potential treatments. We hope that in the future, new drug treatments in individuals might be identified using a similar approach.

Philippa adds, 'I think the challenge is our level of understanding of how this disorder starts, why some women get it and indeed what actually is going on in terms of why this so called lesion can cause the associated problems.'

The elusive 'endometriosis' diagnostic test

Ovarian and deep endometriosis is now increasingly diagnosed by imaging, such as ultrasound and MRI. It is the superficial/peritoneal subtype of the disease that proves the biggest challenge. We think that one of the main reasons that progress has not been made to identify a biomarker that can be used to test for endometriosis is due to the fact that, until now, many studies have been on a small-scale and involved poorly defined populations of women and samples. We are confident that we will see a change in the progress in this area, with the efforts that have been made to improve endometriosis definition. Professor Christian Becker, from the University of Oxford says: 'The average time between the onset of symptoms and a diagnosis of endometriosis ranges between 8–12 years worldwide. Sensitive biomarkers are the key to reduce the time of suffering for millions of women. Despite increasing efforts, no clinically relevant biomarkers for endometriosis exist at the present time. Only large, multi-centre collaborative studies using standardised sample and data collection tools, will enable us to identify and validate biomarkers for a heterogenous condition such as endometriosis.'

Is surgery the best way to treat endometriosis?

The evidence for the benefit of surgery for endometriosis – particularly for improving painful symptoms – is, unfortunately, only based on a small number of studies, and whilst these may be of good quality, they are often studies that include women with a range of the different types of endometriosis rather than specific types.

Dominic Byrne says, 'A lot of basic science is missing, and it's quite hard to get basic science on surgical diseases and operations, because patients and doctors don't welcome random allocation to one treatment or another. Yet that is the purest scientific way of demonstrating one treatment is better than another, so the data we need is quite hard to collect and probably will never fully be achieved. The same with other surgical procedures, so an element of experience drives the knowledge base, rather than pure science driving the knowledge base.'

Nevertheless, if you look at the success rates of surgery performed in endometriosis centres, it is becoming increasingly clear that symptoms associated with deep endometriosis (and probably, ovarian endometriosis) improve with appropriate surgery. It is particularly heartening that, with hindsight, some women even appear to be cured from their endometriosis.

But, we are aware that more and more clinicians are questioning whether 'cutting out', 'burning' or 'lasering' superficial/peritoneal disease is of benefit to women to treat the painful symptoms of endometriosis. There is good evidence to suggest that surgery for superficial/peritoneal disease increases pregnancy rates. Indeed, is it possible surgery for superficial/peritoneal disease may cause more harm than good, and puts women at risk of multiple operations and the complications that these operations could lead to? We need better evidence about whether surgery is the best way to treat this type of endometriosis. And to do so, we come back to the fundamental need to understand why it happens in the first place.

Dominic says, 'It is actually the other end of the spectrum that's slightly more difficult, and that is patients who have lots of symptoms, but when you look inside their pelvis or abdomen you find very little or very limited disease. It is hard to understand what can be the cause of their disease, so that's frustrating. It may be that they have other causes for their pain, and it may be that they have endometriosis in places we haven't even identified, but in terms of treating them, it's relatively unfulfilling on both sides of the relationship. From my point of view, I explain to them that I think the outcome is likely to be little changed if we remove relatively minor endometriosis. Some women don't have the surgery, and some do, and it's about 50/50 who feel there is an improvement. But that's sort of frustrating from a surgical side.'

Raising awareness

We believe that improved awareness of endometriosis will increase the likelihood that it is diagnosed more quickly. Raising the awareness of endometriosis should not 'on paper' be difficult, but it will only be achieved by support from politicians and governments, including investment and well-thought-out strategies to inform the general public and better educate healthcare practitioners at all levels about endometriosis.

Endometriosis UK play an invaluable role in continually highlighting the condition through social media and campaigning for greater acknowledgement and a much better understanding of this common but frequently misunderstood condition.

How does Emma Cox, Chief Executive of Endometriosis UK, feel about the future? 'I am optimistic that we will start to see diagnosis times reducing in the next few years – yes, that's slower than I, and many others, would like, but it is going in the right direction. This will come about through improved GP training and awareness; greater understanding of what's "normal" for the menstrual cycle through education in schools; and, of course, greater public awareness so women know what questions to ask, and aren't dismissed as having "women's issues".'

Our hope for the future

We have witnessed so many unimaginable advances in science and medicine, whether it's technology that now allows us to peer deep into the body and deliver treatment, or the multiple medicines that extend the lives of people. Think of anaesthetics that dull the pain that had long been associated with surgery, and antibiotics and vaccines that have halted communicable diseases. Think also of the announcement, over 15 years ago, that the majority of the human genome had been sequenced, housing the dawn of a new branch of medicine, medical genomics. And don't forget progress in our methods of conducting research, like the advent of the randomised controlled trial which has given researchers an important tool in determining which treatments work, and which do not, bringing in the current era of evidence-based medicine.

So, we think that the state of medicine today is not an endpoint for women with endometriosis but that it marks a new beginning. There is the enticing promise of the next hopeful steps towards, not only a cure for endometriosis, but the means to identify women at risk of the condition and allow early intervention.

Women's hopes

It is appropriate that we leave the last words to be the hopes of the women we interviewed. You might have imagined that all women asked for a cure, or to understand the causes of endometriosis, or even to have a much simpler diagnostic test. But these hopes, whilst very much there, often remained unspoken – women frequently looked far more pragmatically at what would make a difference here and now, to this generation of women suffering, as well as to the future.

These were less about demands on a heavily burdened health system than a plea for acknowledgement, as Sophie says: 'I've been an Endometriosis UK support group leader for three years now, however, it's sad seeing every few months the same questions repeated, the same struggles. I'd really like in the future that endometriosis is more accepted, more known about by professionals, that women are being referred to services a lot quicker than they are now, and that there is help from the beginning.'

Women hope that, with greater awareness and education amongst clinicians, the diagnosis time might be reduced, as Amy tells us: 'I want there to be greater awareness of it, particularly within the healthcare system, obviously with GPs because it is often the first point of call, then obviously in society at large, with employers. That seven and a half years' statistic (average length of time to diagnosis) needs to come right down. I know that it's an invasive, complex disease, so you know it's never going to be one of those things where everyone goes to the doctor and it's immediately diagnosed, but seven and a half years is too long.'

Alongside this, women want to be listened to, particularly when they have hard decisions to make, so that they can own those choices, as Saskia explains: 'I want them to have treatments that they feel okay with, they're not forced upon them but they feel like their choices have been listened to. Even though when you're stuck between a rock and a hard place, when you have a difficult decision to make, you feel okay that you've made a decision by yourself and it's your decision.'

Few of these asks are about expensive interventions – they are mostly about human interactions and understanding. So why has this been hard? We cannot ignore how difficult it is within a complex system to ensure person-centred care takes priority, but we can, as patients and professionals, continue to work together to ensure that we are all working towards the same end: high-quality care, delivered in the right place on a timely basis. This is something that we, as 'health citizens', all need to own.

Women told us the sort of services they want to receive – services that some women are fortunate to receive now, but not all – and the priorities which sometimes seem far off:

'For pain clinics to be more widely available.' – Sophie
'I wish there were more specialist nurses, it would really change many people's lives.' – Lucy

'On a big-picture level, although I think awareness has increased, one of my biggest frustrations is that the

government hasn't taken this seriously enough, there's still not enough investment in research.' – Zoe

'*We need money for research because we need to know what causes this, because until you know what causes it and why it happens and how it happens, you can't find a cure or find out what medications work best to help control it. Now it might be that there is not a cure, it might be that there is medication to control it, but that's fairyland you know, that's not going to happen or I'd be very surprised if it happens.' – Poppy*

Let's hope this is not 'fairyland' – because all women, and all of the women that come after them – deserve better.

Resources

Support and information

Endometriosis UK
www.endometriosis-uk.org
Pelvic Pain Support Network
www.pelvicpain.org.uk
Self Management UK
www.selfmanagementuk.org
The Samaritans
www.samaritans.org

Information and resources

British Society for Gynaecological Endoscopy (for details
of accredited endometriosis centres):
bsge.org.uk/centre
Counselling and Psychotherapy
www.itsgoodtotalk.org.uk
Disability Rights UK
www.disabilityrightsuk.org
Endometriosis.org
www.endometriosis.org

NHS Choices
www.nhs.uk/Conditions/Endometriosis/Pages/Introduction.
aspx

NHS (for NHS England specialised commissioning guideline for deep (severe)/ complex endometriosis):
www.england.nhs.uk/commissioning/wp-content/uploads/
sites/12/2014/04/e10-comp-gynae-endom-0414.pdf

NICE (for guidance on endometriosis):
www.nice.org.uk/guidance/ng73

ESHRE Guideline on Endometriosis
www.eshre.eu/Guidelines-and-Legal/Guidelines/Endometriosis-guideline.aspx

The Pain Toolkit
www.paintoolkit.org

Pelvic, Obstetric and Gynaecological Physiotherapy
pogp.csp.org.uk

Support and information on fertility-related issues

Donor Conception Network
www.dcnetwork.org

The Ectopic Pregnancy Trust
www.ectopic.org.uk

Fertility Friends
www.fertilityfriends.co.uk

Fertility Network UK
fertilitynetworkuk.org

Genesis Research Trust
www.genesisresearchtrust.com

Miscarriage Association
www.miscarriageassociation.org.uk

Support and information on adoption

Adoption UK
www.adoptionuk.org

Information on work-related issues

Equalities and Human Rights Commission
www.equalityhumanrights.com

Glossary

Ablation: surgical term used to mean to destroy or remove tissue.

Adenomyosis: the finding of endometrial-like tissue within the myometrium (muscular wall of the womb).

Adhesions: scar tissue.

BAME: black and minority ethnic.

Barium enema: an X-ray exam that can detect changes or abnormalities in the colon (an enema is the injection of a liquid into your rectum through a small tube).

Biopsy: sample of tissue.

Bilateral salpingo-oopherectomy: removal of both Fallopian tubes and ovaries.

Bladder scan: ultrasound scan to check that your bladder is able to empty completely.

Bowel resection: surgical removal of segment of the bowel loop.

Catheter: tube put into the bladder.

Colonoscopy: camera examination of the colon by means of a flexible tube inserted through the anus (may be done under general anaesthetic but most commonly awake with sedation).

CT scan (computerised tomography scan): special X-ray tests that produce cross-sectional images of the body. Contrast material is sometimes given (either swallowed, injected via an intravenous line or administered by enema) to make it easier to see some structures.

CT intravenous urogram (CT IVU): an examination of the kidneys, ureters and bladder that uses iodinated contrast material injected into veins.

'Down regulation': down regulation is the process of lowering a cell's sensitivity to specific molecules and/or hormones. Drugs used in endometriosis to down regulate the ovaries include GnRH agonists and antagonists.

Dysmenorrhea: period pain.

Dyspareunia: pain with sex.

Ectopic pregnancy: pregnancy implanted outside the uterus (womb), most commonly in the Fallopian tube.

Endometrioma: cyst that occurs on the ovaries with endometriosis, sometimes called a 'chocolate cyst' because it contains old blood which is brown-coloured.

Enema: a procedure in which liquid or gas is injected into the rectum to expel its contents, in order to introduce drugs or permit X-ray imaging.

Embryo: a human offspring during the period from approximately the second to the eighth week after fertilisation (after which it is usually termed a foetus).

Excision: surgical term for cutting away.

Fallopian tubes: the tubes along which the sperm travels from the womb to the ovaries, and in which the egg if fertilised into an embryo and travels back to the womb.

FGM (female genital mutilation): which involves removal of the clitoris and is sometimes known as 'female circumcision', 'cutting' or *sunna, gudniin, halalays, tahur, megrez* or *khitan*. FGM is carried out for various cultural, religious and social reasons. It is illegal in the UK.

GnRH gonadotrophin-releasing hormone agonist/analogue: a type of drug that blocks GnRH receptors. When administered over a long period reduces blood levels of oestrogen and testosterone.

HRT hormone replacement therapy: oestrogen and/or progesterone.

Hysterectomy: surgical removal of the womb.

Hysteroscopy: camera test to allow surgeon to look into the inside of the womb. May be done under general anaesthetic but most commonly done when awake.

IBS (irritable bowel syndrome): a common disorder affecting the colon that causes cramping, abdominal pain, bloating, gas, diarrhoea and constipation.

ICSI (intracytoplasmic sperm injection): a technique of in-vitro fertilisation in which an individual sperm cell is injected into an egg.

IVF (in-vitro fertilisation) a medical procedure whereby an egg is fertilised by sperm outside the body in a laboratory.

Laparoscopy: a camera test under general anaesthetic that allows a surgeon to look inside the pelvis.

Laparotomy: open surgery.

Laser surgery: a type of surgery that uses the cutting power of a laser beam.

MRI magnetic resonance imaging: a technique for producing images of bodily organs by measuring the response of body tissues to high-frequency radio waves when placed in a strong magnetic field.

NICE The National Institute for Health and Care Excellence: provides national guidance and advice to improve health and social care.

Oestrogen: a sex hormone produced by the ovary.

Oopherectomy: removal of the ovary.

Ovary: a female reproductive organ (a woman usually has two) in which eggs are produced, located each side of the womb.

Ovarian cyst: fluid-filled sacs or pockets within or on the surface of an ovary.

Peritoneum: the serous membrane that lines the walls of the abdominal cavity.

Person-centred care: an approach that focuses on the elements of care, support and treatment that matter most to the patient, their family and carers.

Pouch of Douglas: an extension of the peritoneal cavity between the rectum and the back wall of the womb.

Progesterone: a sex hormone produced by the ovary.

Progestins: synthetic forms of progesterone.

Progestogens: the term that describes the body's natural progesterone and synthetic progestins.

Randomised control trial: a study in which people are allocated at random to receive one of several clinical interventions. One of these interventions is the standard of comparison, or 'control'. The control may be a standard practice, a placebo ('sugar pill'), or no intervention at all.

IVP or IVU (intravenous pyelogram or intravenous urogram): an X-ray procedure used to visualise abnormalities of the urinary system, including the kidneys, ureters and bladder.

Sigmoidoscopy: camera examination of the sigmoid colon by means of a flexible tube inserted through the anus. May be done under general anaesthetic but most commonly awake with sedation.

Stoma: an artificial opening made through the skin into the gut.

Transvaginal ultrasound: a type of pelvic ultrasound used by doctors to examine female reproductive organs – 'transvaginal' means 'through the vagina'.

Ultrasound: the creation of a picture called a sonogram by sending sound waves out through a probe.

Ureter: the tube from the kidney to the bladder.

Acknowledgements

We are extremely grateful to all the women, healthcare practitioners and researchers who took the time to share their experiences and views with us. We are particularly indebted to the women – not only those that we interviewed but also those whose stories we know so well and who motivated us to write this book. Without their help, it would not have been possible.

We are heavily indebted to the expertise and dedication of Emma Cox, the Chief Executive of *Endometriosis UK*. Her hard work and commitment to women with endometriosis means that thousands of women across the UK receive much better information and support than they would do otherwise.

Special thanks to Ronnie Grant for his help with the illustrations, as well as everyone who peer reviewed the book prior to publication: Helen McLaughlin, Wendy-Rae Mitchell, Mr Fevzi Shakir, Louise Stanley, Sonya Timms, Emma Tegala, Dr Paul Vinson and Jackie Young.

We must also thank Andrew's partner, our families and friends for supporting our efforts to produce this book. Lastly, thank you to our editor, Emma Owen, Justine Taylor, and everyone from Penguin Random House for their insight, enthusiasm and assistance in producing this book.

Index

stories, how women coped 178–84
superficial/peritoneal endometriosis
xviii, xix, 10, 18, 22, 23, 29, 37,
71, 76–7, 113, 144, 145, 146,
207, 209, 211, 212
support groups 44, 133, 178, 182–4,
215 *see also under individual
group name*
surgery x, xiii, 4, 19, 24–31, 50, 51,
55, 57, 59, 60, 61, 62, 63, 68–95
A&E and 100–1
beyond 87
bowel 78–84
complications 86–7
deep endometriosis and complex
76–8
efficacy of treating endometriosis
with 87–9, 211–13
fertility and 145–6, 149, 151, 159
hysterectomy 89–92
laparoscopic *see* laparoscopic
surgery
menopause and 92–5
types of 72–3
urological 84–6
symptoms ix, x, xiii, xvii–xix, 2–3,
8–9
bladder xviii, 19, 36
bleeding 21–2 *see also* bleeding
bowel xviii, 16–18, 31–3, 35
fatigue 19–21
GP and 102–111
gynaecologist and 111, 114, 116,
117
information on 10–11
pain and symptoms diary 11, 14,
47, 104, 109, 110

pain as 11–16 *see also* pain
treatment of endometriosis focus
on 170–3
types of endometriosis and 22–3

talking 178–9
Thea 18, 55–6, 62–3, 75, 76, 81–2,
188–9, 190, 203
treatments ix, x, xiii, xiv, 49–95
hormone treatments 52–67
pain medications 50–2
route planning 49–50
surgery 68–95
see also care pathways
Triptorelin 61

urological investigations 35–7
urological surgery 84–6

Vicki 91, 104, 174

woman's anatomy, a xxi, 78–9
work and careers 140–1, 186–95,
221
changing career paths 191–3
disability 189–90
employers, dealing with 193–5
flexible working 190–1
sickness absences 186–9
work relationships, managing
140–1

Zoe 2, 11–12, 26–7, 63, 75, 90–1,
119, 135, 137, 139, 156, 157–8,
170, 171, 177, 178, 179, 188,
201–2, 205, 216
Zoladex™ 61, 62–3, 64, 172